ABC of
Spinal Disorders

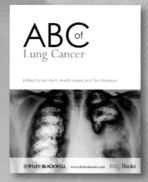
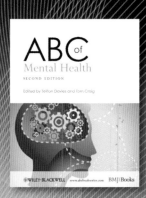
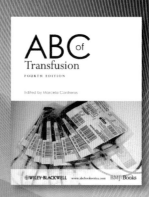
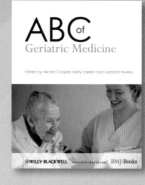
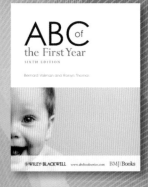
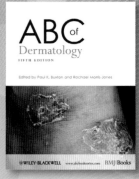

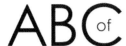

ABC of

Spinal Disorders

EDITED BY

Andrew Clarke

Specialist Registrar, Trauma and Orthopaedics, Royal Devon and Exeter Hospital - Peninsula Deanery, Devon, UK

Alwyn Jones

Consultant Spinal Surgeon, University of Wales Hospital, Cardiff, UK

Michael O'Malley

Consultant Orthopaedic Surgeon, Warrington Hospital, Warrington, UK

Robert McLaren

General Practitioner, London, UK

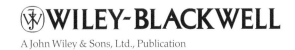

WILEY-BLACKWELL

A John Wiley & Sons, Ltd., Publication

BMJ|Books

This edition first published 2010, © 2010 by Blackwell Publishing Ltd

BMJ Books is an imprint of BMJ Publishing Group Limited, used under licence by Blackwell Publishing which was acquired by John Wiley & Sons in February 2007. Blackwell's publishing programme has been merged with Wiley's global Scientific, Technical and Medical business to form Wiley-Blackwell.

Registered office: John Wiley & Sons Ltd, The Atrium, Southern Gate, Chichester, West Sussex, PO19 8SQ, UK

Editorial offices: 9600 Garsington Road, Oxford, OX4 2DQ, UK
              The Atrium, Southern Gate, Chichester, West Sussex, PO19 8SQ, UK
              111 River Street, Hoboken, NJ 07030-5774, USA

For details of our global editorial offices, for customer services and for information about how to apply for permission to reuse the copyright material in this book please see our website at www.wiley.com/wiley-blackwell

Library of Congress Cataloging-in-Publication Data

ABC of spinal disorders / edited by Andrew Clarke . . . [et al.].
    p. ; cm. – (ABC series)
  Includes bibliographical references index.
  ISBN 978-1-4051-7069-7
  1. Spinal – Diseases – Diagnosis. 2. Spinal – Diseases – Treatment. I. Clarke, Andrew. II. Series: ABC series (Malden, Mass.)
  [DNLM: 1. Spinal Diseases – diagnosis. 2. Spinal Diseases – therapy. 3. Back Pain – physiopathology. 4. Spinal Injuries.
WE 725 A134 2010]
  RD768.A22 2010
  617.4′82 – dc22

                                                                                    2009018583

ISBN: 9781405170697

A catalogue record for this book is available from the British Library

Set in 9.25/12 Minion by Laserwords Private Limited, Chennai, India
Printed and bound in Singapore
1   2010

Contents

Contributors

John R. Andrews
Consultant Spinal Surgeon, Newcastle

Adrian Brown
Physiotherapist, Wales

Richard Brown
Consultant Chiropractor, Gloucestershire

M.P. Caplan
Consultant Radiologist, North Cheshire NHS Trust, Lovely, Warrington

Claire Chambers
General Practitioner, Wiltshire

Daniel Chan
Consultant Spinal Surgeon, Royal Devon and Exeter Hospital, Devon

Andrew Clarke
Specialist Registrar, Trauma and Orthopaedics, Royal Devon and Exeter Hospital - Peninsula Deanery, Devon

Tim Germon
Consultant Spinal Neurosurgeon, Derriford Hospital, Plymouth

Darryl Johnston
Consultant Anaesthetist, Royal Devon and Exeter Hospital, Devon

Anthony T. Helm
Consultant Orthopaedic Surgeon, Royal Preston Hospital, Lancashire

Alwyn Jones
Consultant Spinal Surgeon, University of Wales Hospital, Cardiff

Steve Longworth
General Practitioner and Hospital Specialist, University Hospitals of Leicester, Leicester

Simon MacLean
Specialist Registrar, Trauma and Orthopaedics, New Cross Hospital, Wolverhampton

Walter Llewellyn McKone
Osteopath, London

Elenor McLaren
Clinical Psychologist, Charing Cross Hospital, London

Robert McLaren
General Practitioner, London

Michael O'Malley
Consultant Orthopaedic Surgeon, Warrington Hospital, Warrington

Kate Prince
General Practitioner, VTS, Wessex

Philip Sell
Consultant Orthopaedic Surgeon, University Hospitals of Leicester and Nottingham University Hospitals

R. O. Sundaram
Specialist Registrar, Trauma and Orthopaedics, Mersey Deanery

Rathan Yarlagadda
Specialist Registrar, Trauma and Orthopaedics, Peninsula Deanery

Preface

The spine is a source of significant suffering to patients and much uncertainty to health-care professionals. We hope that this book will provide a framework for managing common spinal problems encountered in everyday practice. We have tried to give as broad an overview as possible, which includes the allied professions of physiotherapy, osteopathy and chiropractics.

CHAPTER 1

Clinical Assessment of the Patient with Back Pain

Philip Sell[1] and Steve Longworth[2]

[1]Consultant Orthopaedic Surgeon, University Hospitals of Leicester & Nottingham University Hospitals, UK
[2]General Practitioner and Hospital Specialist, University Hospitals of Leicester, UK

OVERVIEW

- Back pain is common
- Simple mechanical pain is the most common cause but the differential diagnosis is extensive
- The triage approach facilitates appropriate diagnosis and management

---

The different flag systems are useful tools to support the diagnostic triage. Simple standardized assessment tools may be used to aid diagnosis and assess patient progress.

Introduction

Back pain is the third most common symptom presented to general practitioners after headache and fatigue. While most patients with back pain seen in primary care will have 'simple mechanical back pain', there is a long list of potential diagnoses, some of them serious and life threatening. The concept of diagnostic triage has been developed to facilitate the efficient and effective diagnosis and management of patients presenting with back pain in primary and secondary care.

Diagnostic triage

When we are talking to patients and colleagues it is important to make sure that we are using words in the same way. Confusion frequently arises because of simple misunderstandings (Box 1.1). The clinical assessment should aim to place the patient into one of three diagnostic groups. When taking the history, be alert for flag features (Box 1.2).

Box 1.1 **Some important definitions**
Where is the back?
From the point of view of diagnostic triage 'the back' means 'the low back' or lumbosacral region, defined as the area on the dorsal

---

surface of the body from the bottom of the 12th rib to the gluteal folds (Figure 1.1).

Where is the leg?
In common parlance 'the leg' is frequently used to mean 'the lower limb' but this is anatomically incorrect. In relation to referred and nerve root pain, the leg is the structure between the knee and the ankle; between the hip and the knee is the thigh. There is an analogous situation in the upper limb; the arm is between the shoulder and the elbow, and the forearm is between the elbow and the wrist.

Where is the hip?
Patients frequently refer to the buttock, lateral pelvic area or lateral upper thigh region as 'the hip'. In fact, pain here is often referred back pain. It is instructive to ask the patient to point with a finger to the painful area. Genuine hip pain is usually experienced in the groin and anterior thigh.

What is sciatica?
Sciatica is a misnomer. The pain that we now know to originate from the lumbar nerve roots was originally thought to be due to pressure on the sciatic nerve. The name 'sciatica' persists, even though the pain has nothing to do with the sciatic nerve.

What is pain?
Pain is an unpleasant sensory and emotional experience associated with actual or potential tissue damage or described in terms of such damage.

Source: (International Association for the Study of Pain)

Box 1.2 **Flags in back pain**

Red flags	–	Indicate potential serious pathology
Yellow flags	–	Risk factors for chronicity, the psychosocial barriers to recovery
Orange flags	–	Psychiatric issues in patients with back pain
Blue flags	–	Occupational issues
Black flags	–	Organizational barriers to recovery

ABC of Spinal Disorders. Edited by Andrew Clarke, Alwyn Jones, Michael O'Malley and Robert McLaren.
© 2010 by Blackwell Publishing, ISBN: 978-1-4051-7069-7.

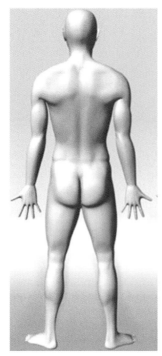

Figure 1.1 Photograph or diagram of the back of the body with the area defined as the back (from the bottom of the 12th ribs to the bottom of the buttocks) shaded in.

Simple mechanical back pain

Simple mechanical back pain accounts for more than 90% of acute episodes of back pain in primary care.

- Onset (first episode) is generally between 20 and 55 years.
- Pain is felt in the lumbosacral region (Figure 1.1). Pain may be **referred** to the buttocks and thighs **but** back pain dominates over limb pain (Box 1.3).

Box 1.3 **Referred pain and root pain**

Referred	Root
Back > limb	Limb > back
Dull ache	Lancinating
Above knee	Below knee (usually)
Unilateral or bilateral	Unilateral
Non-dermatomal	Dermatomal
No aspect (front/back/side) or edge	Aspect and edge
No sensory symptoms	+/− sensory symptoms
No neurological signs	+/− neurological signs
Straight leg raise (SLR) − ? back pain worse	SLR − leg pain worse

---

- Pain is 'mechanical' in nature, i.e. it **varies** with physical activity and posture over time (within and between episodes) and during the examination.
- The quality of the pain and its location within the lumbosacral region are highly variable and frequently unhelpful in diagnosis.
- The patient is systemically well, with no risk factors for serious pathology (see below).

- Prognosis is good with 90% recovery from the acute attack in 6 weeks.

Nerve root pain

Nerve root pain is associated with 5–10% of acute episodes of back pain in primary care.

- Unilateral **leg** pain is present below the knee (but S1 pain is occasionally felt in the buttock/thigh only).
- Leg pain ('lancinating' or shooting pain) dominates over back pain.
- Pain generally radiates to the ankle, foot or toes in a dermatomal distribution.
- Numbness and paraesthesia in the same distribution **may** be present (not always).
- Nerve irritation signs are reduced by straight leg raising (SLR), which worsens the **leg** pain but not the back pain.
- Motor, sensory or reflex change is uniradicular. E.g. S1 nerve root – pain (and sensory symptoms if present) in the buttock, posterior thigh, calf, ankle, sole of foot, with or without weakness of buttock clenching, knee flexion, ankle plantar flexion, with or without diminished or absent ankle reflex.
- Prognosis is excellent with 50% recovery in 6 weeks.

Possible serious pathology (red flags)

Possible serious pathology accounts for less than 1% of back pain in primary care.

- Age of onset is <20 years or first episode occurs in >55 years.
- Violent trauma, e.g. road traffic accident (RTA) or fall from a significant height.
- Systemically unwell; ask about fever, weight loss, anorexia, rigors, malaise and sweats (remember Fever WARMS).
- Non-mechanical pain is constant, progressive, not related to posture/activity and is associated with disturbed sleep, nerve root pain, which switches sides; the pain is not helped at all by simple analgesia.
- History of cancer – lung, breast, prostate, kidney and thyroid are the most common primary sources; back pain may be the *first* presentation of cancer elsewhere with pain from metastases – examine the possible primary sites.
- Systemic steroids (increased risk of osteoporotic vertebral collapse, infection).
- Drug abuse and immunosuppression by disease or drugs (increased risk of infection).
- Anticoagulated (increased risk of spinal bleed/haematoma).
- Persisting severe restriction of lumbar flexion.
- Thoracic pain (often mechanical in young primary care patients, beware older patients).
- Worse on lying down (spinal tumour).
- Widespread (polyradicular) neurology and/or upper motor neuron signs.
- Structural deformity (Figure 1.2).
- If there are suspicious clinical features or the pain has not settled in 6 weeks, review and consider arranging investigations (Box 1.4).

Box 1.4 **Investigations for red flags**

Blood tests

Full blood count
ESR/CRP/plasma viscosity
Renal function tests
Liver function tests
Bone profile
Prostate specific antigen (men)
Immunoglobulin electrophoresis (and urine for Bence Jones protein)

Imaging

Plain X-rays if fracture (e.g. osteoporotic wedge fracture) suspected
Isotope bone scan (if infection or widespread metastases suspected)
MRI scan
CT scan

• *Don't forget* that serious visceral disease may present with back pain – e.g. aortic aneurysm, pancreatic cancer, peptic ulcer, renal disease (cancer, stones, infection).

Examination of the lumbar spine

General observation

General observation is through watching the patients as they walk into the consulting room, looking at their

face (pain behaviour and emotional state)
posture (pain behaviour, sciatic tilt and simian posture of spinal stenosis)
gait (pain behaviour, foot drop, antalgic gait of hip osteoarthritis (OA) and neurological gaits)

Standing (patient undressed)

• Ask the patient to indicate the location of their pain.
• Look for deformity (Figure 1.2).
• Look for any scars.
• Kyphosis – look for compensatory hyperextension of the neck.
• Muscle spasm – palpate for hypertonic paraspinal muscles (they feel solid, not soft).
• Schober's test (McRae's modification) – the *only* validated test in back pain; persistent restriction correlates with significant spinal pathology (Figure 1.3).
• Active lumbar extension/side flexions are not diagnostically informative. Some believe that back pain worse with flexion originates in the disc and that back pain worse with extension comes mainly from the facet joints. There is little supportive evidence.
• Walking on the tiptoes screens for S1 myotome strength.
• Walking on the heels screens for L4/5 myotome strength.
• Romberg's Test – can the patient stand steadily with feet slightly apart and eyes closed? Inability to do so suggests a posterior column lesion.
• Walking heel-to-toe tests cerebellar function.

• Waddell's Tests (Figure 1.4) – If you suspect abnormal illness behaviour, perform vertical skull compression, pseudo rotation of the lumbar spine; pinch a fold of skin over the lumbar area ('ground glass back').

The three other Waddell tests are the flip test (see below) and widespread non-anatomical sensory change in the lower limbs and widespread non-myotomal weakness (often jerky, giving way on isometric testing).

If the patient's symptoms are confined to the back such that there are no limb symptoms, the patient has a normal gait and you do not suspect abnormal illness behaviour, then it is unlikely that examining the lower limbs will contribute any further useful diagnostic information.

Supine

• Exclude the hips – flex the hip and knee to 90 degrees and rotate the hip laterally and medially (in OA hip, medial rotation will be more painful and limited).
• SLR – with the knee fully extended, cup the heel in the hand and slowly raise the limb to 90 degrees; if the test is positive it usually reproduces or exacerbates the pain **in the leg** (not the back) in the first 30 degrees. Flex the knee and the pain in the leg should diminish, allowing further hip flexion with increased leg pain on extending the knee again. If you suspect abnormal illness behaviour and cannot perform the SLR because of pain (often bilaterally restricted and making the back pain worse), ask the patient to sit up while you ostensibly palpate the lumbar spine; if they can sit fully forward with their legs extended while distracted, you have a positive 'flip test' (another Waddell test). The SLR may be limited by hamstring tightness (they will tell you it is stretching in the back of the thigh).
• 'Crossed pain' (i.e. SLR on the asymptomatic side increases the symptoms on the symptomatic side) is pathognomonic of a large disc prolapse. This sign has high specificity but very low sensitivity.
• Isometric muscle strength testing for nerve root dysfunction (you are looking for weakness; CAVEAT; pain may sometimes cause apparent weakness).

N.B. There is considerable overlap between the nerve supply to the muscles and the areas of skin supplied by individual nerve roots in individuals – look for the overall pattern of neurological features.

• Motor

L2 – Resisted hip flexion
L3 – Resisted knee extension
L4 – Resisted ankle dorsiflexion
L5 – Resisted big toe dorsiflexion/ankle eversion
S1 – Resisted ankle plantar flexion

• Sensation

Check light touch/pin prick
L3 – Anterior thigh
L4 – Inner leg

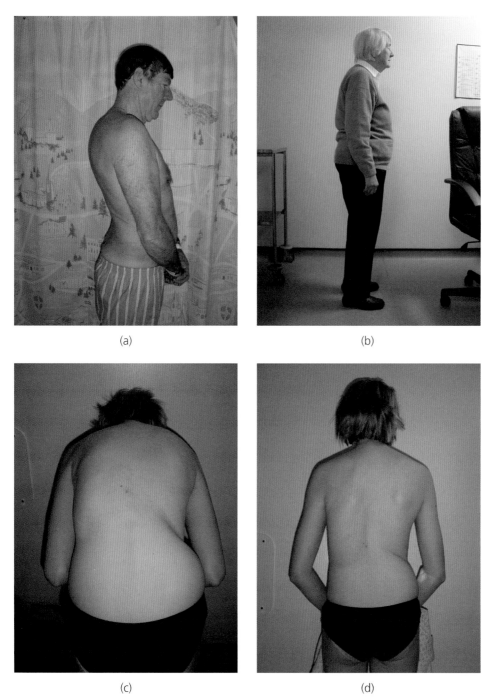

(a)

(b)

(c)

(d)

Figure 1.2 Photographs or diagrams of sciatic tilt, (a) scoliosis, (b) thoracic kyphosis, (c) spondylolisthesis and (d) simian posture of spinal stenosis.

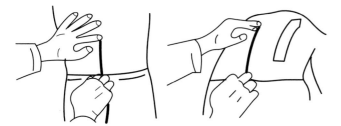

Figure 1.3 Diagram illustrating Schober's test: 'A 10- cm line is marked on the patient, extending from the posterior superior iliac spines towards the head. On forward flexion, this line should increase in length by at least 5 cms.'

L5 – Outer leg/top of foot

S1 – Back of calf, bottom of foot

- Palpation – palpate the pedal pulses to help differentiate vascular and spinal claudication (spinal stenosis)
- Reflexes – knee (L3)

Prone

- Isometric muscle strength testing

  S1 – ask the patient to clench their buttocks tight

  S1 – resisted knee flexion

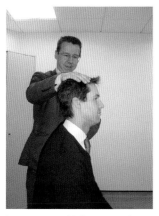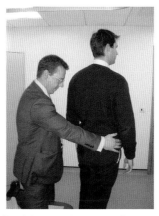

Figure 1.4 Waddell's tests – photographs of doctor and patient to illustrate vertical skull compression, pseudorotation and the ground glass back.

R – How are others **Responding** to your back pain (family, co-workers, boss)?
T – Have you ever had **Time** off work in the past with back pain?
I – **If** you are currently off work when do you expect to return? Ever? What do you feel about your job?
F – **Financial** – time off work causing financial hardship? Any outstanding legal/insurance claims? Receiving benefits (including disabled parking badge)?
I – What **Investigations** have you had so far and what did they show?
C – What are you doing to **Cope** with the back pain?

- Femoral stretch test (L3 nerve root)
  Flex the knee to 90 degrees and lift the knee from the couch – positive if flexion reproduces/exacerbates pain in anterior thigh from L3 nerve root lesion – uncommon
- Reflexes – ankle (S1)

Palpation

Palpation of the lumbar spine is surprisingly unhelpful in reaching a diagnosis, as pain is so poorly localized.

- The step deformity of a spondylolisthesis is typically best felt (and seen) in standing.
- Localized tenderness of the vertebrae is highly sensitive for osteomyelitis, but unfortunately, it has very poor specificity.
- If there is widespread superficial tenderness to palpation (and pinching of skin folds), this is often a feature of abnormal illness behaviour.
- Palpate along the course of the sciatic and peroneal (at the head of the fibula) nerves for lumps. Neuromas of these nerves may cause distal neurological symptoms and signs.

Yellow, orange and blue flags

In patients with back pain that is not settling after 6 weeks, a biopsychosocial assessment should be made. In practice, this means that besides making a search for red flags, a search should also be made for psychosocial, psychiatric and occupational obstacles to recovery (Box 1.5). Chronic pain is often accompanied by depression (Box 1.6). The relationship between chronic pain and depression is complex. Treating the depression decreases pain as well as improves functional status and quality of life.

Box 1.5 **Yellow, orange and blue flags**
Certificate
Interview prompts to elicit psychosocial, psychiatric and occupational obstacles to recovery.

C – What do you understand is the **Cause** of your back pain?
E – Have you **Ever** had any other chronic pain problem (chronic whiplash, irritable bowel syndrome, tension headaches, fibromyalgia, RSI, PMS etc.) and what happened?

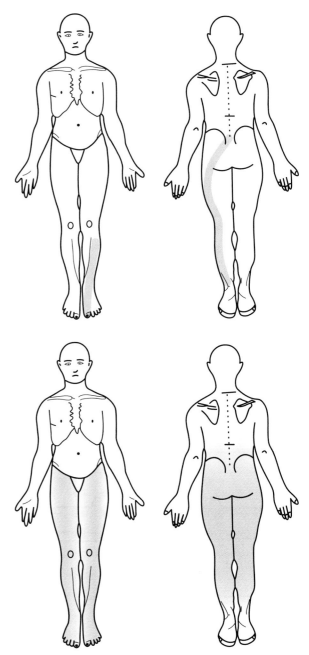

Figure 1.5 Pain drawings; one anatomical, one distressed.

A – **Affective** – some people with long-term pain get low, down or depressed; how is your mood at the moment? (Box 1.6)

T – What have you been **Told** about your back pain by your GP/physiotherapist/osteopath, etc?

E – **Expectations** – what were you hoping we might be able to do?

Box 1.6 **Screening questions for depression**

- Have you often been bothered by feeling down, depressed, or hopeless?
- Have you often had little interest or pleasure in doing things?

When both answers are no, people are unlikely to be depressed, i.e. the screen is highly sensitive, but positive replies to the questions have lower specificity, requiring further questioning from the clinician to confirm the diagnosis. If the answer to either question is 'yes', then a positive response to a third question increases specificity.

- Is this something you would like help with?

Black flags

Organizational factors frequently manifest as barriers to recovery, e.g. long waiting times for outpatient appointments, physiotherapy and imaging tests. These issues frequently emerge when assessing patients with back pain.

Standard assessment tools

These forms are simple and straightforward to complete and a selection can be stapled together and given to the patient to fill in before the consultation. They are helpful diagnostically and can provide useful consecutive measures of pain, disability, somatization and depression during follow-up (Box 1.7).

Box 1.7 **Some standardized back pain assessment tools**

Visual analogue pain scales for back and limb pain
Oswestry Disability Index
Low Back Outcome Score
Roland and Morrison Back Pain Questionnaire
Fear Avoidance Beliefs Questionnaire
Main's Somatic Index
Zung Depression Index
Pain drawing (Figure 1.5)

Further reading

Waddell G. *The Back Pain Revolution*, 2nd edn. Churchill Livingstone, 2004.

CHAPTER 2

Imaging of Spinal Disorders

M.P. Caplan

North Cheshire NHS Trust, Warrington, UK

OVERVIEW

- The principle radiological investigation for spinal disorders has been the radiograph in the past
- Radiographs provide direct evidence of the bony skeletal changes, but only indirect signs of soft tissue abnormalities
- Cross-sectional imaging techniques such as magnetic resonance imaging (MRI) have improved our appreciation of disease in patients with spinal disorders

Indications for imaging

In patients presenting with spinal disorders a relevant history and focused clinical examination will identify the minority of patients requiring imaging. Radiological investigations are appropriate in selected patients to guide treatment and exclude serious underlying pathology.

There is a large range of symptoms related to spinal disorders, but back pain with or without neurological symptoms is the most common presentation, potentially generating large numbers of requests for radiological investigation. Many studies have established that the majority of acute back pain episodes resolve without need for investigation or specialized treatment and there are well-established recommendations regarding the use of imaging based on the available evidence.

Acute spinal pain

Radiographs continue to be performed for acute episodes (less than 6 weeks), but infrequently contribute to the patient's management, unless there is a history of trauma or suspected vertebral insufficiency fracture. Disc herniation is readily demonstrated on MRI scans to confirm the level of disc protrusion and demonstrate compression of neural structures (Figure 2.1). Patients who have a history of trauma, with progressive neurological deficit, at risk of osteoporosis or with 'red flag signs' of suspected

serious underlying pathology (Table 2.1) should be recognized and may require imaging. Patients with suspected cauda equina syndrome should be referred as an emergency to hospital because of the danger of irreversible neurological deficit if not treated promptly. These patients may present with saddle anaesthesia, abnormalities of bowel and bladder control and rapidly progressive motor neurological deficit. MRI scanning is more appropriate as the first radiological investigation for patients presenting with neurological symptoms (radiculopathy, cauda equina syndrome, symptoms of cord compression or myelopathy) or signs of infection. The whole spine can be evaluated and displayed by joining images of the cervical, thoracic and lumbo-sacral levels (Figure 2.2).

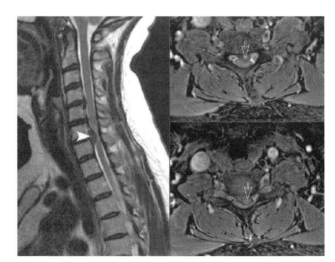

Figure 2.1 Sagittal and axial MRI scans demonstrating a large cervical disc protrusion at C6/7 compressing the spinal cord (arrows).

Table 2.1 Red flag signs.

Age of onset <20 years or >55 years
Fever and unexplained weight loss
Bladder or bowel dysfunction
History of cancer
Progressive neurological deficit
Disturbed gait, saddle anaesthesia

ABC of Spinal Disorders. Edited by Andrew Clarke, Alwyn Jones,
Michael O'Malley and Robert McLaren.
© 2010 by Blackwell Publishing, ISBN: 978-1-4051-7069-7.

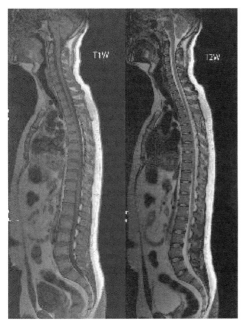

Figure 2.2 Whole spine sagittal T1W and T2W images.

Chronic spinal pain

The majority of patients (85%) have non-specific back pain due to presumed stress on spinal and paraspinal tissues, but with the development of minimally invasive and surgical techniques more patients are being investigated for the cause of pain. MRI is increasingly used as the first imaging study in patients with chronic low back pain to evaluate degenerative disc disease, facet arthrosis and spinal stenosis (Figure 2.3). MRI demonstrates disc dehydration with reduced nucleus pulposus signal on T2 weighting and can identify tears of the disc annulus. Vertebral end-plate changes in bone marrow signal, named *Modic changes* since being first described by Michael Modic in 1988, are frequently seen around degenerate discs and may be referred to in radiology reports. They

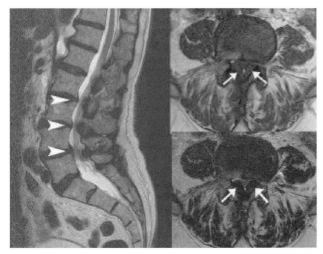

Figure 2.3 Spinal stenosis due to annular disc bulges (arrowheads) and thickening of the ligamentum flavum (arrows).

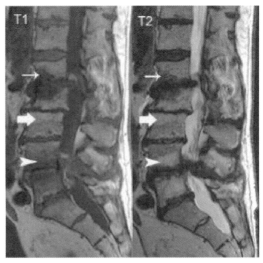

Figure 2.4 Type I (arrowheads), II (large arrow) and III (small arrow) Modic end-plate changes.

are categorized according to the MRI appearances (Figure 2.4), indicating bone marrow oedema (type I), fatty infiltration (type II) or sclerosis (type III).

Spinal trauma

Plain X-rays are indicated as the initial investigation for symptomatic patients, if there is impaired consciousness, or in multiple injuries. Cervical radiographs after whiplash injury to the neck are the most frequently ordered examination for trauma to the spinal column. Standard films include lateral, anteroposterior and odontoid peg views, supplemented by penetrated swimmer views if the cervico-thoracic junction is not adequately demonstrated. If there is localized pain or reduced level of consciousness and high probability of fracture that may not have been seen on the plain films, a computerized tomography (CT) scan is indicated. CT is more sensitive for fracture than radiography and may be used as the first modality in the patient who is obtunded or has multiple injuries. MRI can be used to evaluate spinal cord and ligament injury in patients with a neurological deficit or suspected ligament disruption and instability. Unstable ligamentous injury may occur without fracture and can also be assessed with flexion and extension X-rays in the fully conscious patient.

Radiological techniques

Radiography

The use of radiographs has significantly diminished with development and greater availability of more sophisticated imaging techniques, but still has a role in trauma and demonstration of insufficiency fractures in patients with a relevant history or risk factors. The role of radiographs in excluding serious underlying pathology has clearly been limited by MRI and nuclear medicine, but radiographs may still be requested because access to more appropriate cross-sectional techniques is often limited or subject to

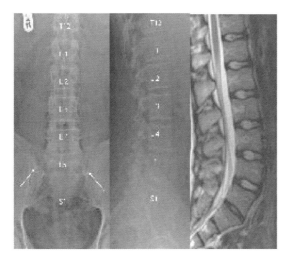

Figure 2.5 A transitional vertebra at the lumbo-sacral junction on X-ray and MRI.

Table 2.2 Contraindications to MRI.

Cardiac pacemakers
Cochlear implants
Some prosthetic heart valves
Some intracerebral aneurysm clips
Nerve stimulators
Ocular metallic foreign bodies

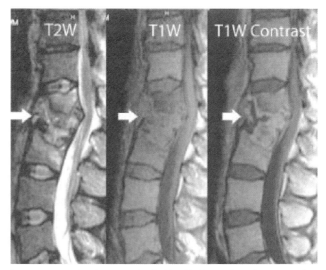

Figure 2.6 MRI showing pyogenic discitis with destruction of T11-12 and the adjacent vertebrae, enhancing after intravenous gadolinium.

significant waiting times. Spondylotic changes secondary to degenerative disc and facet joint disease are common in the normal middle age adult population, increasing with age, and have been likened to observing the prevalence of grey hair. In patients presenting with suspected spinal injury, radiographs are performed to exclude fractures and to guide further imaging strategies. Transitional vertebrae are common at the lumbo-sacral junction and may be suspected on MRI. An anteroposterior radiograph including the thoraco-lumbar and lumbo-sacral junctions may be required prior to surgical intervention to correctly number the lumbar vertebrae (Figure 2.5).

Magnetic resonance imaging

Over the past two decades, MRI has developed into the most accurate imaging tool for the majority of orthopaedic and neurological disorders. A basic understanding of the physics of MRI is helpful, both to have some understanding of its physical basis relevant to safety precautions and to understand the technical terminology of radiological reports.

MRI utilizes the phenomenon of nuclear magnetic resonance to provide contrast between normal tissues and disease. When protons are placed in a very strong magnetic field, they oscillate at a frequency proportionate to the field strength and absorb electromagnetic energy in the form of radio waves, which are at the same frequency of oscillation. They return to a state of equilibrium, releasing radio wave energy that is detected to create the images. The restoration of equilibrium can be measured in the longitudinal plane in T1-weighted (T1W) and the transverse plane in T2-weighted (T2W) sequences. Tissues differ in the rate at which they achieve equilibrium, providing excellent contrast between normal soft tissues and disease processes. Water appears dark on T1W and bright on T2W images.

Normal fat appears bright on most sequences so that many examinations utilize 'fat-suppressed' sequences to make pathology more conspicuous.

Safety concerns with MRI scanning are related to the very strong magnetic field generated by the superconducting electromagnet, so

that there are contraindications in a small proportion of patients (Table 2.2).

It is important to correlate MRI findings with the clinical presentation because disc degeneration and disc prolapses are commonly found in asymptomatic individuals. Disc dehydration, annular bulges and focal protrusions are common findings in the normal adult population and may not be related to the patient's symptoms. MRI provides excellent demonstration of soft tissues of the spine showing disc dehydration, disc herniation, nerve root compression, disc and paraspinal infection and primary or secondary neoplasms. Normal bone marrow signal, with its high fat content in adults, provides excellent contrast to diseases such as vertebral tumours, osteomyelitis and degenerative vertebral end plate changes.

Contrast enhanced MRI may be indicated for evaluation of spinal infection (Figure 2.6), subarachnoid spread of neoplasm or a lesion with the spinal cord or canal, such as a neoplasm or inflammation (myelitis). Contrast is also used in the post-operative lumbar spine to differentiate recurrent disc protrusion from scar (epidural fibrosis).

Nuclear medicine

Isotope bone scans utilize technetium 99m bound to diphosphonate and taken up in normal bone. Areas of increased activity indicate active bone lesions due to increased osteoblastic activity. The isotope is given intravenously and the patient returns in about

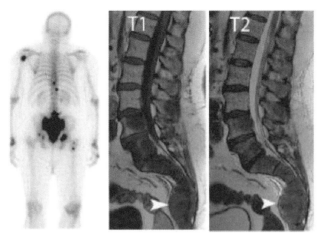

Figure 2.7 Isotope bone scan and MRI showing metastatic disease, with a large deposit in the sacrum (arrowhead).

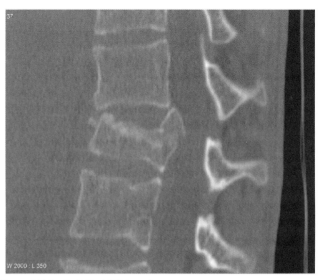

Figure 2.8 Sagittal CT of T12 burst fracture.

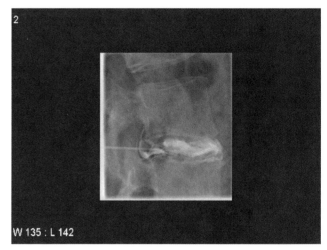

Figure 2.9 Lumbar discogram.

3 hours for imaging of the skeleton. Early phase dynamic and blood pool images of specific regions may be taken to demonstrate hypervascular and inflammatory lesions. Delayed scans after about 3 hours demonstrate 'hot spots', indicating areas of increased activity due to increased osteoblastic activity.

Bone scans are commonly used to determine if a known lesion is solitary or multiple and are highly sensitive in demonstration of metastases (Figure 2.7) and other active lesions such as an osteoblastoma.

Computerized tomography

Computerized tomography (CT) utilizes a rotating X-ray tube to provide cross-sectional images. Current scanners use movement of the patient table during continuous tube rotation (spiral or helical CT) to enable contiguous slice acquisition and allow multi-planar reconstructions (MPR) in the sagittal, coronal or oblique planes. CT provides excellent detail of the skeleton and is most often used in spinal conditions to identify and characterize vertebral fractures (Figure 2.8). In patients for whom MRI is contraindicated, a CT myelogram may be performed to demonstrate the thecal sac and nerve root sheaths. CT has the disadvantage of high exposure to ionizing radiation and is inferior to MRI in demonstrating soft tissue abnormality.

Discography

A discogram is a specialized invasive procedure during which a needle is guided into one or more intervertebral discs to determine if there is structural damage and if the disc is causing pain. Annular tears are demonstrated by leakage of contrast from the nucleus pulposus (Figure 2.9) and a pain provocation test during injection provides evidence that the painful symptoms are related to the level examined. It is usually performed prior to spinal fusion or disc replacement.

Conclusion

Radiological investigations have an essential role in the investigation of spinal disorders, invaluable in demonstrating a wide variety of abnormalities and in the exclusion of serious pathology. The excellent sensitivity of MRI in demonstrating disc degeneration, disc herniation, spinal infection, neoplasms and spinal stenosis in selected patients has revolutionized the diagnostic pathway, but must be correlated with clinical findings.

Further reading

The Royal College of Radiologists. *Making the Best Use of Clinical Radiological Services. Referral Guidelines.* The Royal College of Radiologists, London, 2007.

CHAPTER 3

The Paediatric Spine

Alwyn Jones

University Hospital of Wales, Cardiff, UK

OVERVIEW

- Back pain is common and increases with age and is usually benign in origin
- Scoliosis is normally conservatively treated but only occasionally requires operative treatment depending on the severity
- The history is crucial in paediatric conditions, which directs the investigation

---

The evaluation of a child with a spinal problem requires a carefully planned approach. An efficient and accurate method of assessment is therefore needed to ensure that nothing is missed.

Most children present with pain, suspected deformity or other problems uncovered during unrelated investigations, such as a chest radiograph showing a thoracic hemivertebra.

Some patients may present, while still in utero, with a congenital spinal abnormality detected on the 20 weeks' anomaly scan and therefore, it is obvious that you will be treating both the parent and the unborn or born child when you assess a paediatric patient.

Back pain

The prevalence of back pain in children and adolescents ranges between 11 and 50%. The occurrence of back pain before 7 years of age is rare and increases to 10% by the age of 10 years and rises to 50% by the age of 15 years. By late adolescence the rate approaches that of adulthood, namely, 60 to 80% but only 2 to 15% will seek medical advice.

Studies from spinal units indicate that in only 50 to 66% a diagnosis is made. Spondylolysis and spondylisthesis are the most common causes of back pain in children but tumours can be found in 5 to 10% of cases. In children below the age of 10 years discitis and tumour are the most common, whereas in more than 10-year-olds spondylolysis, spondylolisthesis and Scheuermann's disease are most common. If a diagnosis cannot be made it is best to re-evaluate after a period of observation.

Painful scoliosis describes symptoms and signs and not a diagnosis. Severe pain is uncommon in idiopathic scoliosis although up to 25% can have a mild pain. Pain interfering with daily activities warrants further evaluation. Backpack use has been linked to back pain but there are no scientific studies to confirm an association; but guidelines suggest the use of both shoulders with a lighter load (Table 3.1).

Children of parents who exhibit chronic back pain problems are at higher risk of similar complaints. There is a genetic predisposition to back pain, and psychological causes also exist in children and adolescents, but at a lower prevalence than in the adult population.

Paediatric spinal history

It is essential to interview the parent as well as the child to maximize the completeness of the assessment. It should be done in an unhurried and thorough manner.

Pain should be classified as mechanical if brought on by activity and relieved by rest, or non-mechanical if unchanged by activity. Mechanical pain lies in the realm of the spinal surgeon. A complete assessment of the pain is required including duration, precipitating factors, site, systemic symptoms, night pain and treatment received. If daily activities are affected then it requires a thorough evaluation.

In relation to deformity assessment, peri-natal history, duration, progression, pain, menarche, family history and associated congenital or neurological symptoms are necessary.

Table 3.1 Guide to the causes of back pain.

Disorders	Neoplastic disorders
Spondylolysis/spondylolisthesis	Benign (osteoid osteoma, osteoblastoma,
Scheuermann's disease	aneurismal bone cyst)
Painful scoliosis	Malignant (leukaemia, lymphoma,
	sarcoma)
Traumatic	
Disc herniation	**Psychosomatic back pain**
Vertebral fracture	
Overuse (sprains)	
Inflammatory/infective	
Discitis	
Vertebral osteomyelitis	
Rheumatological disorders	

ABC of Spinal Disorders. Edited by Andrew Clarke, Alwyn Jones, Michael O'Malley and Robert McLaren.
© 2010 by Blackwell Publishing, ISBN: 978-1-4051-7069-7.

Family history is important in idiopathic scoliosis, inflammatory conditions and hereditary neurological diseases.

Congenital deformities need to be assessed in regard to associated conditions including cardiac, renal, anorectal as well as intra-canal conditions such as syringomyelia, diastematomyelia and tumours.

In deformity following trauma, pain is usually a significant issue as well as a functional change.

Examination

Begin with gait, and trunk and limbs for symmetry. Asymmetry should raise concern. Skin abnormalities such as hairy patches, dimples or lipomas should signal underlying dysraphism. Common anterior chest wall abnormalities are pectus carinatum and excavatum. Percussion of the spine and sacroiliac joints can suggest infection if tender. Pelvic obliquity and loss of lumbar lordosis can be assessed in standing position. A scoliometer can be used to assess topographical abnormality, and Adams forward bend test is also useful. Twenty percent of adolescents may have truncal asymmetry on forward bend test but fewer than 2% may have an underlying scoliosis. A scoliometer reading of 7 degrees should be an indication for radiographic evaluation of the whole spine as shown in Figure 3.1.

Increased kyphotic deformity in the sagittal plane will be easier when assessed in the forward bent position. An increased kyphosis would suggest either Scheuermann's disease, congenital kyphosis or scoliosis with underlying intraspinal pathology.

In the sitting position the neck can be formally assessed for movements and deformity. Torticollis is a sign of several conditions ranging from congenital muscular torticollis, syndromic conditions, inflammatory and atlanto-axial rotatory abnormalities. Upper limb function can be best assessed in the sitting position.

Finally in the examination the child is supine and the abdomen can be assessed to include abdominal reflexes. Asymmetry suggests underlying spinal cord abnormality. Range of motion of the joints, limb size and length and neurological assessment is performed.

Investigations

Plain radiographs allow visualization of the vertebrae, disc spaces, destructive processes and deformity in the sagittal and coronal planes. Every child with persisting back pain should have a radiograph of that area of the spine. Spondylolysis (pars defect) can be detected in only a third of patients.

Radiographs should establish a diagnosis suspected from the history and examination. Idiopathic scoliosis is diagnosed when a 10-degree or greater curve is seen with rotation. A full-length posterior–anterior (PA) film is performed to minimize radiation exposure to the thyroid and breasts. The superior pelvis is visualized to allow Risser grading of skeletal maturity. This is important in the assessment of curve progression. Riser grade 0 is prepubertal, grades I and II signify beginning of rapid growth and grades III and IV decreasing growth (Figure 3.2).

The Cobb angle can be identified by the angle subtended by a line drawn above the proximal most tilted vertebra and a line drawn below the most distal tilted (end) vertebra (Figure 3.3).

Spondylolysis and spondylolisthesis are found in approximately 6% of the population. The isthmic type where there is a pars defect can be seen on the lateral radiograph, particularly in a listhetic patient. Pars defects can be seen on an oblique film, with the collar of the 'Scottie dog' but now we tend to further investigate this with computerized tomograph (CT) or magnetic resonance imaging (MRI). In spondylolisthesis, the degree of slip can be classified on the percentage slippage of the vertebra upon the vertebra below; grade I, 1 to 25%; grade II, 26 to 50%; grade III, 51 to 75% and grade IV, 76 to 100%. Spondyloptosis denotes where the vertebral displacement is beyond 100%.

CT scans are useful for three-dimensional views of congenital spinal abnormalities, fractures and for bone tumours. Spondylolysis can be assessed with regard to age as well as fracture gap and orientation. CT scanning is used to assess fusion post-operatively

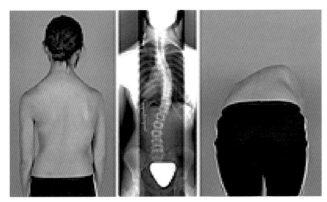

Figure 3.1 Adam's forward bend test. (Left) As the patient bends over, the examiner looks from behind and from the side, horizontally along the contour of the back. (Right) A rotational deformity known as a *rib hump* (arrow) can be easily identified.

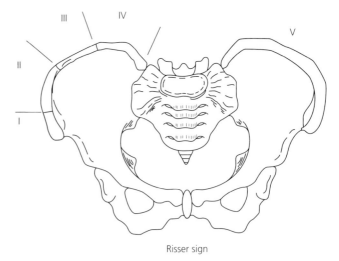

Risser sign

Figure 3.2 Risser grades 0 to V. Grading is based on the degree of bony fusion of the iliac apophysis, from grade 0 (no ossification) to grade V (complete bony fusion).

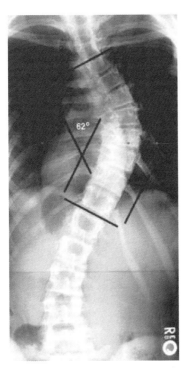

Figure 3.3 The Cobb method of measuring the degree of scoliosis. The physician chooses the most tilted vertebrae above and below the apex of the curve. The angle between intersecting lines drawn perpendicular to the top of the superior vertebrae and the bottom of the inferior vertebrae is the Cobb angle (here, 62 degrees).

and to check on the position of metalwork. Cervical anatomy can be clarified with CT films, especially at the craniocervical junction.

MRI is the gold standard for intraspinal and paraspinal soft tissue abnormalities. Knowledge of normal anatomy is essential in the interpretation of MRI. Imaging the very young child can be difficult for compliance and often requires a general anaesthetic, as well as their specific anatomical differences. The conus alters in level with age, and up to 25% of adolescents will have radiological evidence of disc degeneration.

MRI will confirm a diagnosis of discitis, epidural abscess, disc herniation, spinal cord tumour as well as other congenital abnormalities.

Bone scans are used in patients with infection, fractures, tumours and spondylolysis. Technetium is the most commonly used in patients with spinal disorders to assess level of bone turnover. Pathological areas of heightened activity are associated with infection, tumours and fracture. It can be a good tool in the assessment of a child with a painful scoliosis where the pain cannot be localized.

Single photon emission computed tomogram (SPECT) is CT of conventional bone scans. It improves diagnostic ability of bone scanning by separating bony structures and localizing anatomical areas. Approximately 25% of lesions seen on SPECT will be seen on plain films and normal bone scan will only show about 50%.

Spinal deformity

Deformity can be classified in the coronal plane as scoliosis and in the sagittal plane as a kyphosis. Scoliosis has a rotational element which is visualized as the rib or loin hump.

Scoliosis is classified into idiopathic (80%), congenital, neuromuscular (neuropathic or myopathic) and syndromic on the basis of its aetiology. Intra- and extra-spinal tumours must also be considered.

Idiopathic scoliosis is classified on the basis of its age of onset as early (<5 years) and late (>5 years). The prevalence of idiopathic scoliosis with a curve greater than 10 degrees ranges from 0.5 to 3%. Larger curves above 30 degrees range from 1.5 to 3 per 1000. Obviously, the earlier the onset, the greater the risk of severe thoracic deformity. Risk factors for progression are gender, curve location and magnitude as well as skeletal immaturity (Risser grade). Curves above T12 are more likely to progress than lumbar curves.

Curves of less than 30 degrees tend not to progress into adulthood but curves between 50 and 75 degrees do so markedly. This progression occurs at a rate of approximately 1 degree per year.

Treatment involves monitoring as curves less than 20 degrees require no treatment, whereas curves above this may require bracing or operative management.

Bracing is reserved for curves between 25 and 40 degrees in skeletally immature patients (Risser <3). Braces do not tend to reduce the curve but hold it at the level of initiation of bracing. Some curves can progress after braces are removed.

Surgical treatment is dependent on the age of onset as growing systems are used in the early onset group. There are several systems on the market, which involve repetitive operations and a definitive fusion in adolescence. In the older age-group definitive fusion can be performed from the posterior or anterior or through a combined approach depending on the curve magnitude and location.

In congenital scoliosis, hemi-vertebrectomy or convex hemi-epiphysiodesis may be performed to correct the deformity.

Kyphosis tends to refer to Scheuermann's disease (vertebral wedging of 5 degrees), congenital abnormality or postural round back.

Scheuermann's disease can occur in the thoracic spine or less commonly in the lumbar spine. Pain can occur in 50% of adolescents.

Physiotherapy benefits postural runback. Surgical treatment is reserved for curves greater than 65 degrees in Scheuermann's disease.

Further reading

Literature

Weinstein, SL. Idiopathic scoliosis: natural history. *Spine* 1986; **11**: 780–783.

Web sites

www.sauk.org.uk
www.srs.org

CHAPTER 4

The Cervical Spine

Tim Germon

Derriford Hospital, Plymouth, UK

OVERVIEW

- Listen to the patient – the most important factor in making a diagnosis is what the patient tells you
- The earliest manifestation of cervical myelopathy may be gait disturbance and falls
- The best test to rule out treatable pathology is an MRI scan. This needs to be interpreted in the context of the patients' problem
- Symptoms resulting from nerve root or spinal cord compression can respond well to surgery
- There is little evidence for the efficacy of surgery or injection therapy in the treatment of neck pain in the absence of radicular symptoms

---

Introduction

Cervical pathology may manifest itself with neurological symptoms or pain or a combination of both.

In common with all spinal symptoms, it is important to distinguish those that are likely to progress without intervention from those that are likely to resolve spontaneously. It is also important to recognize that symptoms of pain and neural involvement may be remote from the cervical spine.

Pathology may primarily affect musculoskeletal or neurological components of the cervical spine or a combination of the two. Whatever the likely cause, severe and progressive pain, neurological deficit or deformity should trigger urgent investigation.

Presentation

Patients with cervical pathology may present with pain, neurological symptoms or both. The most common pathology is degenerative disease, and symptoms are unlikely to be rapidly progressive. However, in common with all disease of the spine, if symptoms are rapidly progressive urgent investigation is warranted.

ABC of Spinal Disorders. Edited by Andrew Clarke, Alwyn Jones,
Michael O'Malley and Robert McLaren.
© 2010 by Blackwell Publishing, ISBN: 978-1-4051-7069-7.

History

Although the majority of patients will have symptoms as a result of degenerative disease it is important to be aware of the potential for the underlying cause being trauma, infection or tumour. 'Red flags' have been described to try and help identify those patients who are likely to be harbouring a potentially serious or progressive condition. It is also important to be aware that other diseases are associated with specific spinal problems, for example, rheumatoid arthritis and ankylosing spondylitis.

Neurological symptoms

The patient may have symptoms of radiculopathy, myelopathy or a combination of both, myeloradiculopathy. The patient's history is by far the most important factor in the diagnostic process (Figure 4.1).

Symptoms of myelopathy

The cardinal symptoms of cervical myelopathy are unsteady gait and clumsy hands. However, early symptoms are often subtle and non-specific. The lower limbs are usually affected before the upper limbs but this is not always the case. Cervical myelopathy is a common cause of falls in the elderly but in the absence of other symptoms and signs, diagnosis may be delayed.

Fine motor tasks may be difficult although these symptoms have often developed insidiously and may not be volunteered by the patient. They will often find it difficult to perform tasks such as doing up buttons, writing or knitting.

As the condition progresses the patient becomes more disabled with an increasingly spastic gait and difficulty with day-to-day tasks such as feeding and personal hygiene. They may complain that their legs jump spontaneously at night or that they suffer electric-shock-like sensations in their spine or limbs.

Sphincter disturbance is common, although frank incontinence is rare except in association with severe and rapid onset cord compression.

Sensory disturbance is common. Numbness affects the upper and lower limbs, starting distally and spreading proximally. They may complain of heat or cold in the affected limbs. Occasionally there may be painful dysaesthesia.

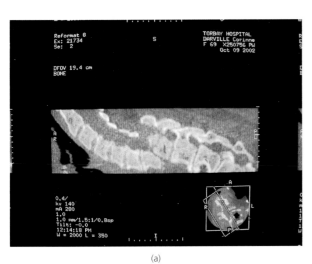
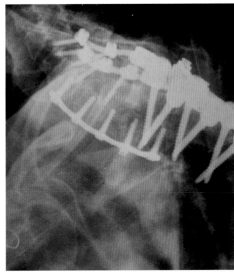

(a)　　　　　　　　　　　　　　　(b)

Figure 4.1 This lady fell backwards on a chair, striking her head on a patio. She had immediate neck and bilateral arm pain. She attended the local A&E department where, on the basis of an inadequate X-ray, she was reassured and prescribed physiotherapy. Despite protesting, 'My chin never used to be on my chest', it took 3 months to obtain a CT scan that confirmed the diagnosis of C7/T1 fracture dislocation. The deformity was corrected and fixed internally with anterior and posterior surgery.

The majority of cervical myelopathy is a result of degenerative disease causing pressure on the spinal cord and is usually not painful. However, it may be associated with radicular pain from a compressed nerve root or with neck pain.

The majority of myelopathy associated with spondylosis will progress in a stepwise manner. Some cases will stabilize and a very few may spontaneously improve. Myelopathy associated with instability of the vertebral column (tumour, trauma and infection) is usually more rapidly progressive and needs to be addressed with more urgency.

Signs of myelopathy

Seeing the patient walk is an essential part of the examination that is often omitted, particularly if the patient is in a hospital bed. It is possible to have apparently normal lower limb on neurological testing of a patient supine but the patient cannot walk. The characteristic spastic broad-based gait may be observed. Sometimes, severe spasticity results in the ankles being held in a plantar flexed position, which appears at a glance to be a foot drop.

There may be the classic signs of cord compression, increased tone, hyper-reflexia, clonus, Hoffman's sign and other signs of myelopathy.

Cervical cord compression can result in lower motor neuron dysfunction as a result of compression of the motor neuron cell bodies that lie within the spinal cord at the compressed level. This can result in the 'myelopathic hand' (Figure 4.2) and may be confused with other causes of clawing.

Cranial nerve examination may suggest a brain stem rather than spinal cord problem. However, it is worth remembering that the trigeminal nucleus does descend into the cervical cord, and this may explain facial symptoms that are sometimes associated with brachalgia.

Symptoms of radiculopathy

Pain is the most common symptom of pressure on a nerve root. The pain may describe a classic dermatomal distribution and be associated with paraesthesia or other sensory or motor disturbance. In these circumstances it is relatively straight-forward to identify nerve root compression as the likely cause of the symptoms. However, pain from a compressed nerve root may not correspond to the classical description. Arm pain is usually associated with neck pain, shoulder girdle pain and often headaches. The diagnosis becomes more difficult when more axial pain is not clearly associated with symptoms affecting the upper limb.

Occasionally, the main feature of a compressive cervical radiculopathy can be the motor or sensory disturbance with very little pain although this is unusual.

Signs of radiculopathy

The classic signs of a lower motor neuron lesion – fasciculation, wasting weakness and hyporeflexia – may be present. They may have a dermatomal pattern of sensory disturbance. If the patient has myeloradiculopathy, the examination will reveal mixed signs.

Pain

As with low back pain, the challenge in patients presenting with neck pain is to establish a diagnosis. Patients may present with classic brachalgia, with pain radiating in the textbook distribution of a particular dermatome. However, pain provocation studies and clinical experience suggest that this is the exception rather than the rule.

Pain as a consequence of nerve root compression responds well to decompression and thus, nerve root compression is an important diagnosis to consider.

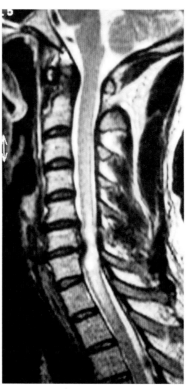

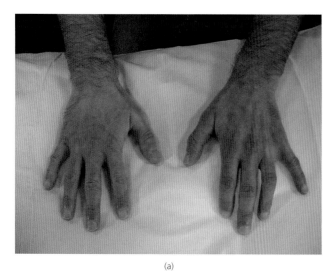

(a)   (b)

Figure 4.2 This man presented with unsteady gait and clumsy hands. Examination revealed upper motor neuron signs along with wasting and clawing. His MRI scan revealed severe cord compression with associated high signal change within the cord.

Neck pain associated with arm pain in a dermatomal distribution is often straight-forward. Neck pain without clear radicular symptoms is more difficult to diagnose. Sometimes the pain distribution may be characteristic. For example, pain radiating over the occiput is suggestive of greater occipital nerve pathology and in the context of rheumatoid arthritis is highly suggestive of atlanto-axial instability. However, occipital headache is commonly seen in association with cervical nerve root compression at other levels.

Neck pain is a common complaint and in common with all spinal pathology; it is important to try and distinguish those likely to harbour 'serious spinal pathology' and those that may be amenable to surgical intervention. Often a diagnosis cannot be made with certainty. In those patients who have neck pain in whom radiological findings cannot be correlated with symptoms (e.g. those with no radicular symptoms), there is no scientific evidence that any surgery or injection therapy is efficacious.

Examination

Patients may have an obvious deformity or they may exhibit very little movement, walking into the consultation with the head held rigid. They may have a gait suggestive of myelopathy and may be using a walking aid. Examination of the neck should determine range of motion, deformity or areas of tenderness.

Standard neurological examination of the upper and lower limbs should be performed. Particular attention should be paid to the distribution of upper or lower motor neuron signs. It can be difficult to distinguish between a spinal nerve root problem and a peripheral nerve problem. It can also be difficult to distinguish between symptoms emanating from the neck and those emanating from the shoulder, and formal examination of the shoulder may be indicated. The lower limbs should be examined for signs of myelopathy.

Radiological investigation

Plain radiographs can be useful in the evaluation of the cervical spine but their utility is limited. The most common finding is of degenerative change, which becomes universal with increasing age. They give no direct information about the spinal cord and nerve roots and their ability to influence management is far inferior to magnetic resonance imaging (MRI).

They do demonstrate alignment, degenerative change, most but not all fractures and destructive processes such as spondylodiscitis and tumour. The problem is that a considerable amount of bone destruction has to occur before it will be detected on a plain X-ray. Flexion–extension views may be indicated if there are specific reasons to suspect abnormal movement but they only rarely change management decisions in degenerative conditions. If they are performed, false-negative results as a consequence of pain inhibition should be guarded against.

MRI scanning has transformed the investigation of the spine. It demonstrates the spinal cord and nerve roots and is sensitive to pathological process in the vertebral column. However, all investigations may have both false-positive and false-negative results. A

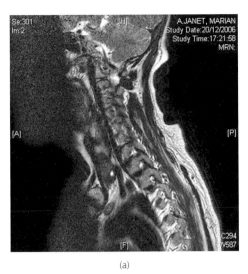
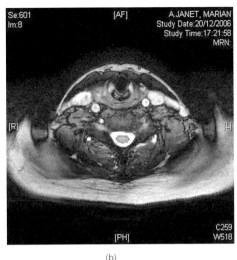

(a)   (b)

Figure 4.3 This lady presented with severe persistent pain in a classical C7 distribution. Her MRI scan was reported as normal. In fact, there was a fragment of disc in the C6-C7 exit foramina, which accounted for her symptoms. Decompressive surgery resulted in complete resolution of her pain.

scan may be reported as not offering an explanation of a patient's symptoms. If this is the case but the patient has persistent disabling symptoms, the scans should be reviewed (Figure 4.3).

Computerized tomographic (CT) scan is used diagnostically to rule out or further characterize a fracture that may be responsible for the patient's symptoms.

Myelography is a sensitive test for spinal cord and nerve root compression. It is mainly used when MRI scan is contraindicated.

Bone scan is sensitive to changes in spinal metabolic activity. With the advent of MRI its value is generally limited to determining the extent of bone disease such as myeloma.

Neurophysiology

Neuropysiological investigations can be a useful adjunct, especially in trying to distinguish between nerve entrapment syndromes and radiculopathy. Nerve Conduction Tests is diagnostic of brachial neuritis.

Blood tests

Blood tests are rarely helpful in making a diagnosis when a patient presents with a spinal problem. However, they are essential in the assessment of a patient who potentially has a systemic problem either in terms of the underlying disease process or suitability for surgical intervention.

Management

Non-operative management

In common with back pain and sciatica, most neck pain and brachalgia due to an acute disc prolapse will often improve with time. However, nerve root compression as a result of osteophyte formation is less likely to resolve spontaneously. Thus, in the first instance, most patients can be managed with analgesia and advice to keep as active as they comfortably can. A short period (48 hours) of rest may be helpful but the disadvantages of longer periods probably outweigh any benefit. Commonly used analgesics including opiates may be helpful. However, often these agents may not be particularly helpful for nerve root pain and agents such as gabapentin, pregabalin, amitriptyline and nortryptilline are certainly worth a trial. Since the response to these agents is idiosyncratic, both in terms of therapeutic and unwanted effect, it is worth exploring various options for an individual patient.

In patients who have already suffered pain for sometime or those who have had recurrent episodes there should be a low threshold for early imaging.

It is clearly important to exclude 'red flags' in the history and examination. With particular regard to the cervical spine it should be remembered that patients whose cervical spine is completely fused as a result of ankylosing spondylitis or degenerative disease are at risk of unstable pathological fractures that can be hard to identify. If there appears to be a discrepancy between the patient's symptoms and the radiological findings, it is safest to assume that the diagnosis remains in doubt and that the patient may be harbouring a potentially unstable spine. Neurological deficit in the context of trauma (even minor trauma) signifies instability of the spinal column until proved otherwise.

The evaluation of physical therapies is difficult. Without a diagnosis it is difficult to understand the rationale of many physical therapies or prove that they achieve what they claim to. It seems reasonable to empirically suggest isometric exercises in the acute phase when movement to maintain muscle function is painful, and introduce more dynamic exercises in the recovery phase.

For patients with progressive or persistent disabling symptoms management depends on the diagnosis. By far, the best diagnostic test is an MRI scan. This investigation should be requested in all patients with persistent and/or disabling symptoms but it is important that the scan is interpreted by an experienced reporter with a focus on the patient's complaint. Once a diagnosis is made it may be possible to discuss specific treatment.

Operative management

The principles of surgical management are to decompress the neural structures and to restore and maintain alignment of the spine. There is a good chance of both improved pain and function following decompression of the nerve roots and spinal cord, even in patients with advanced neurological symptoms.

Although decompressing the neural elements is often the primary objective, this cannot be safely undertaken without considering the impact of the surgical procedure on spinal stability. If the spinal column is already unstable, or is likely to be rendered unstable by the decompressive procedure then it should be accompanied by stabilization and fusion. Despite this, the patient will often have greater mobility as a consequence of improved pain.

Most spinal surgical objectives can be achieved by employing either an anterior or a posterior approach to the surgical target. The approach employed will be dictated by a combination of the pathology being addressed and the surgeon's preference. Occasionally a combined anterior and posterior approach is required.

Potential complications common to all spinal procedures are spinal cord or nerve root damage and cerebrospinal fluid (CSF) leak. Other potential complications are specific to the particular procedure being undertaken and the approach employed. Clearly, the decision to proceed with surgery should follow discussion of the potential risks and benefits of surgical intervention.

Pathology

Causes of myelopathy and radiculopathy

1. *Extra-dural cord compression*: Degenerative disease of the vertebral column comprises the vast majority of cases. Other pathology includes tumours of the spinal column, of which metastatic disease is by far the most common, infection, trauma and rheumatoid.

2. *Intra-dural extra-medullary cord compression*: Unusual – generally the result of a benign tumour.

3. *Intra-medullary disorders*: Rare – pathology includes tumours or inflammatory conditions.

Differential diagnosis

Radiculopathy

Peripheral nerve entrapment syndromes
Shoulder joint pathology
Thoracic outlet syndrome
Brachial neuritis

Myelopathy

Gait disturbance – normal pressure hydrocephalus (NPH), cerebellar disease, spinal stenosis of thoracic or lumbar spine
Peripheral neuropathy
Guillain-Barre syndrome

Further reading

Carragee, Eugene J., Hurwitz, Eric L., Cheng, Ivan *et al.* Treatment of neck pain: injections and surgical interventions: results of the bone and joint decade 2000–2010 task force on neck pain and its associated disorders [best evidence on assessment and intervention for neck pain]. *Spine* 2008; **33** (4S Suppl.15): S153–S169.

Clarke CR *et al.*, The Cervical Spine Research Society Editorial Committee. *The Cervical Spine*. Lippincott Williams & Wilkins, Philadelphia, 2004.

Slipman CW, Plastaras CT, Palmitier RA, Huston CW, Sterenfeld EB. Symptom provocation of fluoroscopically guided cervical nerve root stimulation: are dynatomal maps identical to dermatomal maps? *Spine* 1998; **23** (20): 2235–2242.

CHAPTER 5

Back Pain

Simon MacLean[1], Claire Chambers[2] and Andrew Clarke[3]

[1]Trauma and Orthopaedics, New Cross Hospital, Wolverhampton, UK
[2]General Practitioner, Wiltshire, UK
[3]Royal Devon and Exeter Hospital - Peninsula Deanery, Devon, UK

OVERVIEW

- It is common
- It is rarely serious
- Staying active promotes faster recovery
- It is a psychosocial phenomenon as well as physical
- Early management reduces disability

The problem with back pain

Back pain affects everybody at some point in their life. Most back pain is self-limiting, short-lived and not because of a serious or often identifiable pathological process. However, it remains to be one of the most enigmatic 'conditions' that confronts health-care professionals. Back pain represents very complex social and psychological problems in association with an anatomical one. In itself, it is not a disease but is a major cause of disability.

The first step for the health-care professional is triaging the serious pathology from the patients presenting with back pain. Then, a successful therapeutic relationship needs to be created with the patients suffering non-specific back pain, in order to overcome their affliction (Table 5.1).

The epidemiology of back pain

The Office of National Statistics (ONS) performed a survey in 1998. They found that 40% of adults reported back pain lasting more than 1 day in the last 12 months. Fifteen percent of these people had been in pain throughout the entire year. Forty percent of sufferers had seen their general practitioner and 10% had visited a complimentary medicine practitioner (Table 5.2).

During the decade 1983 to 1993, there was a fivefold increase in outpatients reporting for back pain. Furthermore, there was a doubling of social security benefits paid during that time for back-related disorders. Between 1988 and 1998, a study reported

Table 5.1 Risk factors for non-specific back pain and chronicity.

	Occurrence	Chronicity
Individual	• Age • Gender • Smoking • General health	• Obesity • Education level • High levels of pain/disability • Unemployment
Psychosocial factors	• Stress • Pain behaviour • Depression • Cognitive function	• Distress • Depression • Somatization • Long duration of pain • Fear-avoidance behaviour
Occupational factors	• Manual handling • Monotonous tasks • Control at work • Job dissatisfaction • Social support • Night shifts • Bending and twisting	• Job dissatisfaction • Lifting for most of the day

(Abridged from Manek NJ and MacGregor AJ. Epidemiology of back disorders: prevalence, risk factors and prognosis. *Curr Opin Rheumatol* 2005; **17**(2):134–140.)

Table 5.2 Back pain and the National Health Service (NHS) in 1 year.

Population prevalence	16,500,000
Consulting GP	3,000,000–7,000,000
Outpatients	1,600,000
Inpatients	100,000
Surgery	24,000

GP, general practitioner.
(Abridged from Bandolier 19 – 147.)

an increase of 12.7% in back pain in the United Kingdom. This was mostly due to less disabling back pain. The researchers concluded that the increase was due to changes in attitude and behaviour. The estimated costs to the United Kingdom from back pain are more than £6,000,000,000 per year.

The aetiology of back pain

There are a myriad of causes of back pain. The first sub-division is between pain arising from the spinal column and pain arising elsewhere (Figure 5.1).

ABC of Spinal Disorders. Edited by Andrew Clarke, Alwyn Jones, Michael O'Malley and Robert McLaren.
© 2010 by Blackwell Publishing, ISBN: 978-1-4051-7069-7.

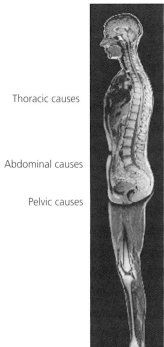

Figure 5.1 Aetiology of non-spinal back pain.

Thoracic causes

Abdominal causes

Pelvic causes

Vascular

Inflammatory

Infectious

Neoplastic

Table 5.3 Broad classification of spinal causes of low back pain and their relative frequency.

Type of pain	Frequency
Non-specific	85–95%
Sciatic/radicular symptoms	5%
Specific (red flags)	1–2%

The second sub-division is into acute and chronic back pain. The changeover is at 6 months. The third sub-division is into one of the three groups in Table 5.3, as this dictates management.

Back pain due to specific pathological conditions will be discussed in other chapters. The remainder of this chapter aims to explore 'non-specific' back pain in greater detail, as this represents the vast majority of back pain.

Non-specific back pain

Once all serious pathologies have been excluded by history, examination and investigations, where appropriate, 'non-specific' or mechanical back pain is the only description possible.

This is an unsatisfactory diagnosis or label for both the patient and the clinician.

Non-organic causes of low back pain need exploring. By applying Waddell's signs (Table 5.4), non-organic back pain can be identified and appropriately dealt with.

Healthy patients may have one or two positive Waddell's signs. Three or more positive signs predicts poor outcome following treatment.

Table 5.4 Waddell's signs.

Waddell's signs
- Pain in non-anatomical distribution
- Pain out of proportion to stimulus
- Exaggerated pain behaviour

Perform four benign tests to assess
- Skin roll test – gently roll loose skin of lower back
- Twist test – gently rotate patient's torso at the hips
- Head compression test – apply small load to top of head
- Flip test – test straight leg raise when seated and supine

Table 5.5 Yellow flags.

- Belief that back pain is harmful or potentially very disabling
- Fear avoidance behaviour and reduced activity levels
- Low moods and withdrawal from social interactions
- Reliant on passive treatments rather than active participation

Psychosocial aspects of back pain need to be explored as well, because they play a very significant part in the disability brought about by this condition. In fact, some view them as barriers to recovery. Table 5.5 highlights these so-called yellow flags.

Combining all patients with non-specific low back pain into one group does not provide a patho-anatomical cause or help to target subsequent therapy. A recent study suggested that in the primary care setting, patients are already being divided into sub-groups by the assessing clinician. Further studies have highlighted that treating all mechanical back pain as a homogenous group is flawed and that it is a heterogeneous entity.

In addition to the heterogeneity of mechanical back pain, the use of clinical reasoning along the 'Medical Model' has been challenged. The absence of a well-defined patho-anatomical reason for the mechanical back pain should not stand in the way of starting treatment. Indeed, the use of the 'Signs and Symptoms Model' advocates planning therapy on the basis of pattern recognition and deductive reasoning.

The classification of non-specific low back pain

No agreed classification system exists for non-specific low back pain. This is because of differences between clinicians in their beliefs. There is much interest in creating a classification, as this could lead to improved outcomes for patients.

Ideally, there needs to be a combination of the history related by the patient to quantify the impairment along with the clinical examination. Then the clinician must judge the severity. Dunn and Croft studied the use of a single question about 'bothersomeness' of back pain to patients. They found that people with very bothersome mechanical back pain at initial assessment had increased risk of work absence and health-care use in the following 6 months.

Currently, practitioners employ a variety of ways to pick their way through back pain. All the methods used involve elements of clinical patterns, response to interventions and risk factors for delayed recovery.

Of specific note in the literature are the works of Delitto and Fritz. Delitto's work identified seven groups of patients. Each group had specific examination findings, and subsequent targeted treatment. Fritz, in partnership with Delitto, performed a randomized trial comparing the use of the classification-based therapy against clinical practice guidelines. They found that the classification-based approach improved disability at 4 weeks.

However, one common theme runs through these attempts to classify mechanical back pain and that is the examination of the patient. Indeed, Mackenzie's classification in 1979 consisted of derangement, dysfunction and posture, followed by sub-classification.

They all try to relate factors that provoke the pain to the spinal structures that are being loaded at that time. Hence, crudely condensed, flexion loads the disc and anterior structures, whereas, extension loads the posterior elements. But, the debate rages on as to the anatomical origin of the pain. Thus, classifying mechanical back pain needs to be more than just a hunt for the pain generator.

Prognosis of non-specific low back pain

Non-specific low back pain is viewed as a benign and self-limiting disorder. However, evidence is accruing that the long-term course of the pain and functional recovery are not as favourable as thought to be.

An Office of Population Censuses and Surveys (OPCS) survey of primary care consultations found that one-third were for patients with back pain who had been pain-free for the last 12 months, one-third for a recurrence within that year and the final third for a persistent problem.

Epidemiological data regarding outcomes is not robust. One study reported that the key prognostic factor was the duration of the current episode. Their second finding was that having a paid job greatly influenced functional recovery. Other work has found that pain characteristics and perception of general health at baseline were prognostic.

Management of non-specific low back pain

The aim of the clinician is to triage the patient's complaint. Once serious pathologies have been eliminated, the process of support begins. Initially, this should be advice, encouragement and analgesia. It is important to accentuate the 'Green Lights' (Tables 5.6 and 5.7). As back pain is such a multi-dimensional issue, clinicians need to engage the patient into taking control of their own recovery. The patient guide from New Zealand (see web links) provides an excellent basis for patient-centric management.

Table 5.6   Green lights.

- Stay active
- Continue normal activities
- Stay positive
- Take medication if necessary
- Manipulation can help in the first month

Table 5.7   Algorithm for low back pain triage.

Visit	Aim	Strategy
First	Diagnostic triage	Red flags – urgent referral
	Symptomatic relief	Nerve root pain – referral
	Prevent disability	Analgesia
		Green lights
1 Week	Clinical reassessment	Green lights
		Physical therapy
4 Weeks	Clinical reassessment	Active rehabilitation
	Psychosocial assessment	Yellow flags – referral
6 Weeks	Clinical reassessment	Secondary referral

Recalcitrant mechanical back pain warrants referral to a spinal service.

Back pain and spinal surgeons

Spinal surgery is provided by neurosurgeons and orthopaedic surgeons in the United Kingdom. Within both groups there are varying beliefs as to the causes and the treatments of mechanical back pain.

To simplify things, there are two broad camps – surgeons who believe in surgical solutions for mechanical back pain and surgeons who do not. There are many weighty tomes written promoting each course of action. Hence, the discussion is too vast for this book.

Further reading

Literature

Deyo R, Rainville J, Kent D *et al*. What can the history and physical examination tell us about low back pain? *JAMA*, 1992; **268**(6): 760–765.

Roland M, Waddell G, Moffett JK *et al*. *The Back Book Norwich*: The Stationery Office, Norwich, UK, 1996.

Web sites

www.nice.org.uk
www.nzgg.org.nz
www.rcgp.org.uk
www.workingbackscotland.com

CHAPTER 6

Sciatica, Stenosis and Spondylolisthesis

Anthony T. Helm[1], *R. O. Sundaram*[2] *and Michael O'Malley*[3]

[1]Royal Preston Hospital, Lancashire, UK
[2]Trauma and Orthopaedics, Mersey Deanery, UK
[3]Warrington Hospital, Warrington, UK

OVERVIEW

- Sciatica is most commonly due to posterior herniation of the nucleus portion of an intervertebral disc

- Cauda equina syndrome is a surgical emergency and requires immediate referral

- Most patients with sciatica can be managed non-surgically

- Spinal stenosis refers to narrowing of the spinal canal, producing sensory and motor symptoms (numbness, pins and needles, pain and weakness) in the legs

- Spinal stenosis is a differential diagnosis in patients with claudication

- Spondylolisthesis refers to a vertebra slipping forward or backward on the vertebra below

- It typically presents in adolescents who are keen sportsmen or gymnasts (isthmic type) or in the older population with a stenotic picture (degenerative type)

Sciatica

Introduction

The life-time risk of a disc herniation is approximately 13 to 40% and the mean age group is between 20 and 40 years. Cauda equina syndrome occurs in 2% of patients with a herniated disc. The majority of disc herniations occur in the lumbar spine; disc herniation of the thoracic spine is extremely rare.

Aetiology and pathogenesis

Degenerative changes within the nucleus pulposus and annulus fibrosus begin from the age of 20 to 30 and cause them to become more fibrotic. This results in the intervertebral disc becoming stiffer and less resistant to deformation. This can lead to a tear of the annulus fibrosus and protrusion of the nucleus pulposus into the spinal canal. Tears in the peripheral annulus fibrosus can also result in back pain. A herniated disc may occur without any

exacerbating factors, or they can occur following an increase in the intra-discal pressure such as when lifting a heavy object.

Radiculopathy

Protrusion of the nucleus pulposus into the spinal canal may irritate a nerve root by direct compression. The most common level of disc herniation is the L4-L5 disc, followed by the L5-S1 disc. Herniations of other discs occur less frequently. The commonest direction of herniation is posterolateral.

History and examination

Patients may often complain of back pain when trying to lift a heavy object followed by severe leg pain and numbness or weakness in the distribution of the affected nerve root. The leg pain, commonly known as sciatica but better described as radiculopathy, usually radiates from the back and follows the dermatomal distribution of the affected nerve root. Patients are very often specific about the pain. Patients can also complain of leg pain without any back pain. The leg pain is the most disabling symptom and this is exacerbated by positions where the spine is flexed, such as when sitting or driving. Standing straight or flat bed rest often improves the leg pain. Enquiry regarding the patient's bladder and bowel function is mandatory. Table 6.1 shows the signs that patients may experience according to the level of the corresponding disc herniation. Ankle and knee reflexes may be absent. Straight leg raising can strongly exacerbate the pain in disc herniations compressing the L4, L5 or S1 nerve roots.

Investigations and treatment

Patients should be initially managed with strong analgesia and physiotherapy for mobilization. Admission to hospital for sciatica is rarely necessary. In 70 to 90% of patients who present with their

ABC of Spinal Disorders. Edited by Andrew Clarke, Alwyn Jones,
Michael O'Malley and Robert McLaren.
© 2010 by Blackwell Publishing, ISBN: 978-1-4051-7069-7.

Table 6.1 Lumbar disc prolapse: signs and symptoms by level.

Level	Sensory	Motor	Reflex
L4	Medial shin	Ankle dorsiflexion	Knee jerk
L5	Lateral shin, dorsum of foot	Great toe dorsiflexion	–
S1	Lateral border of foot	Ankle plantarflexion	Ankle jerk

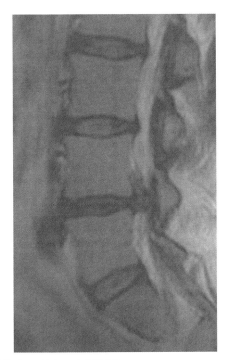

Figure 6.1 Prolapsed intervertebral disc.

first episode of sciatica, their pain usually settles down by 3 months. In 90% of these patients their symptoms do not relapse. Of the 10% of patients whose symptoms relapse, 90% will settle down by 3 months. However in these 10%, up to 50% can experience a further relapse. Patients who experience a third episode of sciatica nearly always go on to have further relapses. If symptoms have not settled by 6 weeks of conservative treatment, a surgical referral is of benefit. An early surgical referral is required if there is progressive neurology or cauda equina syndrome. A magnetic resonance imaging (MRI) scan (Figure 6.1) is the investigation of choice to identify which level the disc herniation has occurred at. Targeted epidural steroid injections can provide excellent relief of symptoms. In the absence of objective weakness that is progressive, MRIs are often used as a first-line intervention, before any surgical procedure. Discectomy is the surgical treatment to remove the part of the nucleus pulposus that is compressing the nerve root.

Table 6.2 Aetiology of spinal stenosis.

Congenital	Acquired
'Trefoil'-shaped canal	Prolapsed intervertebral disc
Achondroplasia	Facet joint hypertrophy
Other skeletal dysplasias	Hypertrophy of ligamentum flavum
Spinal deformity	Degenerative scoliosis
–	Trauma

Cauda equina

Cauda equina syndrome is a true emergency. It is rare, and if surgery is a possibility, requires urgent onward referral to a spinal surgery service for assessment.

The clinical diagnosis can be difficult. Key features relate to bladder and bowel function, along with perineal sensation. The only way to confirm a suspected case is to perform an urgent MRI scan. The patient is then referred to the treating spinal surgeon for subsequent management.

Spinal stenosis

Introduction

Spinal stenosis is defined as any condition that results in narrowing of the spinal canal or foramina.

Aetiology

Most of the causes of spinal stenosis are degenerative in nature. The causes of spinal stenosis are summarized in Table 6.2. When the spinal canal is narrowed by any cause, there is less available space for the thecal sac, which contains the nerve roots, resulting in symptoms of back pain (from the degeneration in the back) and nerve root compromise, which are often exacerbated by activity (Figure 6.2).

Clinical features

The incidence of spinal stenosis increases with age. The patient is usually older than 50 years. The principal complaint is of leg symptoms that are brought on with or exacerbated by exercise and

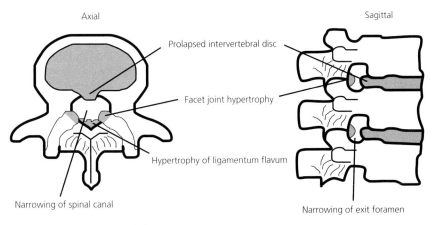

Figure 6.2 Spinal stenosis pathology.

relieved with rest. The leg pain can mimic vascular claudication but a careful history will differentiate the diagnoses. As a rule, the pain of vascular claudication is made worse by walking uphill as the calf muscles are working harder, whereas the pain of spinal stenosis is said to be less when walking uphill because of the larger space available for the spinal nerves when the patient adopts a slightly flexed posture. The symptoms of leg pain and/or radiculopathy are often superimposed on a long history of back pain, reflecting this condition's degenerative nature.

During examination, one should look for evidence of degenerative spinal disease, such as localized tenderness and reduced spinal movements. A neurological examination of the legs is often normal with the patient at rest. If there are symptoms of claudication, a thorough vascular examination of the lower limbs should be performed.

Investigations

The gold standard investigation when spinal stenosis is suspected clinically is a magnetic resonance scan. This can assess the degree of spinal stenosis and also identify the level(s) affected, along with any specific impingement of exiting nerve roots. Figure 6.3 shows a T2 axial image through an area of spinal stenosis.

Treatment

The treatment of spinal stenosis can be broadly divided as non-surgical and surgical.

Non-surgical treatment consists of lifestyle modifications such as losing weight and avoiding exacerbating factors. Physical therapy can help in relief of symptoms, along with adequate analgesia. Epidural injections of local anaesthetic and steroid can also be used. These can be targeted or general injections into the epidural space such as a caudal or lumbar epidural.

Patients who fail conservative therapies can be considered for decompressive surgery, which may be accompanied by fusion. Recent developments include inter-spinous process distraction devices to increase the space within the spinal canal.

Spondylolisthesis

Spondylolisthesis is the slipping of one vertebra on another. It is a common problem, and has an incidence of about 6% in the general population. However, only a small proportion of patients become symptomatic because of spondylolisthesis.

Aetiology

The underlying problem in most spondylolisthesis is that the pars inter-articularis is not normal. When one vertebral body slides forward on another, the nerves can become compressed in the canal and back pain can be caused because of the abnormal mechanics of the back trying to hold the spine together. A deficiency of the pars inter-articularis, also known as a *spondylolysis*, is most often seen in adolescents who are keen sportsmen or gymnasts. A spondylolisthesis can also be acquired through degenerative spinal disease when weakness of the supporting ligaments allows forward slippage of the vertebra. It is very rarely due to acute trauma.

Clinical features

The patient presents with low back pain, exacerbated by exercise. In some cases there will be symptoms of radiculopathy with altered sensation or referred pain in a dermatomal distribution. Adolescents with the 'spondylolysis' or stress fracture of the pars often have tight hamstrings.

Investigations

A plain lateral view of the lumbar spine will often show spondylolisthesis (Figure 6.4). Classically, the pars defect is seen more easily with an oblique view, giving the typical appearance of the 'Scottie dog with a broken neck' (Figure 6.5). Magnetic resonance scanning is indicated if the X-ray does not show spondylolisthesis when it is clinically suspected, when there are radicular symptoms or if surgical fusion of the spine is planned. Additionally, a standing lateral X-ray of the spine is very useful, to assess movement at the spondylolisthesis. This helps to determine whether there is a dynamic element to the slip.

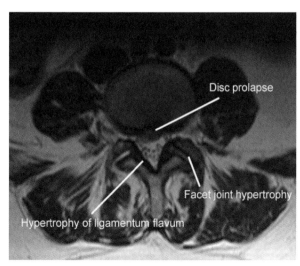

Figure 6.3 Spinal stenosis (MRI).

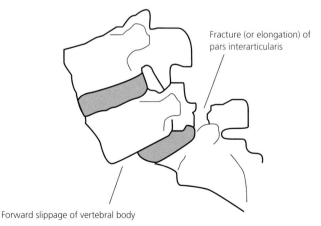

Figure 6.4 Spondylolisthesis.

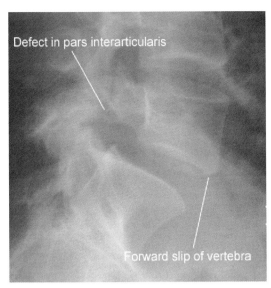

Figure 6.5 Spondylolisthesis (X-ray).

Treatment

Initial treatment is supportive. In athletic adolescents with the lytic spondylolistheis, analgesics and activity limitation are helpful initially. This can be followed by physiotherapy to strengthen the supportive musculature. If this fails to provide adequate relief, then an injection of local anaesthetic into the pars defect is useful to assess how much pain is due to the defect itself and to give an indication of what kind of surgery is required to alleviate the symptoms. Surgery is only indicated for disabling pain or severe radicular symptoms not responding to conservative treatment. Surgery is aimed at stabilizing the spine and, if required, decompression of affected nerve roots.

In patients with degenerative spondylolisthesis, it is imperative to ascertain the main complaint. It can be back pain, stenotic type leg pain, radicular type leg pain or any combination. The slip is unlikely to progress. However, even if it does, this may not correlate with the symptoms of the patient. Therefore, assiduous assessment and the use of targeted injections play a large role in the management of degenerative spondylolisthesis. Surgery can then be planned if required to address the key complaints of the afflicted.

Further reading

Atlas Steven J, Keller Robert B, Wu Yen A *et al.* Long-term outcomes of surgical and nonsurgical management of lumbar spinal stenosis: 8 to 10 year results from the main lumbar spine study. *Spine* 2005; **30**(8): 936–943.

www.dartmouth.edu/sport-trial/publications.htm (This provides publications on the outcomes for sciatica, spodylolistheses and spinal stenosis.)

CHAPTER 7

Tumours, Infection and Inflammation

Rathan Yarlagadda[1] and Daniel Chan[2]

[1] Trauma and Orthopaedics, Peninsula Deanery, UK
[2] Royal Devon and Exeter Hospital, Devon, UK

OVERVIEW

- The commonest neoplasm of the spine is metastasis
- Pain is usually the presenting complaint, neurology is a late symptom.
- MRI is the investigation of choice and early spinal consult is advocated by NICE.
- Infections often present with no systemic symptoms and diagnosis can be difficult, look for risk factors.
- Appropriate antibiotics are the treatment of choice for infection in the spine.
- Inflammatory arthropathy includes rheumatoid arthritis, ankylosing spondylitis, etc.
- Many patients with rheumatoid arthritis and radiographic changes are asymptomatic.
- Spinal fractures in patients with ankylosing spondylitis are easily missed and must be actively looked for.

Primary and metastatic tumours of the spine

The most common neoplastic condition affecting the spine is skeletal metastasis. The most common site of metastatic disease is in the thoracolumbar region (70%). The lumbar and sacral spine accounts for a further 20% and the cervical spine 10%.

Primary bone tumours are rare (0.4% of all tumours). There is a larger incidence in the sacral and cervical area as opposed to the lumbar and thoracic spine.

Presentation

Pain is the commonest presenting complaint for patients with spinal malignancy. This is usually of gradual onset. It can be unrelenting, non-mechanical and worse at night. The pain can become radicular as neural compression occurs.

Acute onset of back pain could be due to a pathological fracture, especially if the patient has a known history of malignancy.

ABC of Spinal Disorders. Edited by Andrew Clarke, Alwyn Jones, Michael O'Malley and Robert McLaren.
© 2010 by Blackwell Publishing, ISBN: 978-1-4051-7069-7.

Neurological symptoms are usually seen with a late presentation. The presence of radicular pain may help in localizing the tumour level. A patient presenting with progressive or rapid neurological deterioration will need urgent assessment.

The patient may also have general symptoms including weight loss, fatigue, anorexia, haemoptysis, hematuria, malena and hematemisis. Always ask for a history of smoking.

Examination

A standard examination of the spine should be performed with a full neurological assessment. The presence of localized tenderness may point to the site of pathology.

Always search for the primary lesion. Examine the prostate, chest, breasts, abdomen, thyroid and lymphatic system.

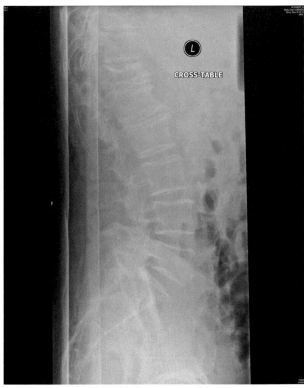

Figure 7.1 X-ray appearances of malignant collapse of T12.

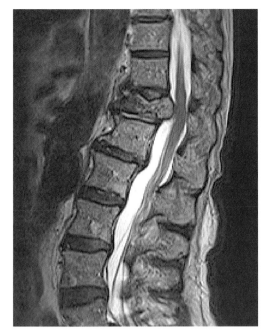

Figure 7.2 MRI appearances of tumour of case in Figure 7.1.

Table 7.1 Primary malignant tumours that affect the spine.

Type of tumour	Treatment
Ewing's sarcoma	Chemotherapy, surgery +/− postoperative radiotherapy
Osteosarcoma	Chemotherapy, surgery and postoperative chemotherapy
Chondrosarcomas	Surgery (not chemo- or radiosensitive)

Investigations

Plain X-rays will help identify up to 80% of benign spinal tumours as well as a significant proportion of primary and metastatic carcinomas. Early metastatic lesions may not be picked up on radiographs (Figure 7.1).

Magnetic resonance imaging (MRI) is the imaging technique of choice for the evaluation of primary and metastatic disease of the spine. MRI is very sensitive and specific for the assessment of metastatic disease. It also helps in differentiating between tumour and infection (Figure 7.2).

A technetium-99m scan is useful for screening patients with a known malignancy. Patients with lung, breast, prostate and kidney or thyroid carcinomas should undergo a bone scan as a part of their initial screening. A biopsy is a requirement for the pre-operative workup of the patient. It should be performed in specialist centers with the site of biopsy decided by the surgeons responsible for the further treatment of the patient.

Benign tumours

Benign tumours are not as common as malignant ones. The patient's age and location are important prognostic indicators. Most tumours tend to be malignant in patients older than 21. In general, tumours involving the posterior elements tend to be benign.

Primary tumours

The three primary malignant tumours that affect the spine are osteosarcoma, chondrosarcoma and Ewing's sarcoma (Table 7.1).

Metastatic tumours

Metastatic disease is the commonest tumour of the spine. The aims of treatment are to control pain, restore neurological function, restore stability and prevent pathological fracture.

The management of metastatic spinal disease is multi-disciplinary including pain control, steroids, chemotherapy, radiotherapy and surgery.

Spinal metastasis presents with pain and/or neurology. Back pain in metastatic disease arises from two causes:

- Direct invasion of bone
- Loss of spinal stability.

Radiotherapy is good for relieving pain caused by the direct invasion of bone by tumour, as long as there is no associated spinal instability.

Percutaneous vertebroplasty is an option for patients with mechanical pain following a pathological fracture. Here, the vertebral body is percutaneously injected with a uni- or bi-pedicular injection of bone cement.

Paralysis can result either from bony compression secondary to a burst fracture or direct epidural compression. A rapid onset paralysis may be associated with a vascular incident to the cord leading to ischemia. This tends to have a poorer prognosis.

High-dose dexamethasone has been shown to be beneficial in improving ambulation in malignant spinal cord compression. However, the gastrointestinal complications associated with large doses of steroids should be considered and in patients with profound deficit, steroids may not be indicated. Always discuss with your local spinal surgeon before starting a patient on steroids.

Infection

Untreated spinal infections may result in deformity and neurological sequelae. With the development of antibiotics and modern methods of surgical management these complications are now uncommon.

Infections of the spine usually present with back pain, often without systemic upset. These infections can result from hematogenous spread from distant sites such as the urinary tract, local spread from adjacent tissues that are infected and from direct inoculation during spinal procedures such as discography.

The most common pathogen is *Staphylococcus aureus* (*S. aureus*) accounting for up to 50% in some reported series. Mycobacterium tuberculosis (TB) is on the rise as a common non-pyogenic cause of infection.

Presentation

The onset is often insidious. Pain is the most common presenting complaint, and is gradual in onset and non-specific. Later stages may be associated with night pain. Constitutional symptoms of

Table 7.2 Risk factors for spinal infection.

Diabetes
Urinary tract instrumentation
Previous spinal surgery
Pre-existing infection: UTI, URTI, etc.
Malignancy
HIV
IV drug abuse
Pre-existing paraplegia
Gunshot wounds

UTI, urinary tract infection; URTI, upper respiratory tract infection;
HIV, human immunodeficiency virus; IV, intravenous.

infection such as fever, night sweats, anorexia, and fatigue and, occasionally for chronic infections, weight loss may be present.

Deformity tends to be a late presentation as are neurological signs. The presence of neurological signs often indicates an epidural infection. Always look for the risk factors for spinal infections (Table 7.2).

The presentation in children tends to be non-specific, with the main complaint sometimes only being general symptoms of malaise and fever, not spinal pain. The child may refuse to weight-bear and may occasionally present with a non-structural scoliosis.

Investigations

The baseline investigations such as erythrocyte sedimentation rate (ESR), C-reactive protein (CRP) and full blood count (FBC) should be performed if a spinal infection is suspected. ESR tends to remain high in chronic infections such as tuberculosis. CRP rapidly returns to normal under appropriate treatment and thus is a good measure of the effectiveness of the treatment given.

Blood cultures should be taken in a search for the causative organism and must be taken before the commencement of any antibiotic therapy.

The radiographic features of infection include the narrowing of disc space, irregularity of the endplates, defects in subchondral bone and sclerosis.

Normal X-rays do not rule out infection. Late features include body collapse, deformity and fusion (Figure 7.3).

The examination of choice in infection is an MRI scan of the spine (Figure 7.4). Bone scans can be used as well, especially in patients in whom an MRI is contraindicated.

Once the diagnosis of infection is confirmed then the responsible organism needs to be found. Blood cultures may help but are positive in only 50% of the patients. Often a tissue diagnosis is required; biopsy is performed using either a percutaneous or an open technique.

Treatment

Treatment of spinal infection requires a combined effort of the spinal surgeon, the microbiologists and the radiologists. Every effort must be made to find the causative organism prior to starting antibiotic therapy. Only if the patient is acutely unwell can broad-spectrum antibiotics be started to cover the most likely causative organism with the guidance of the microbiologists.

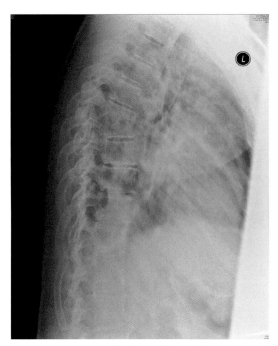

Figure 7.3 X-ray appearances of infection affecting thoracic spine and disc space.

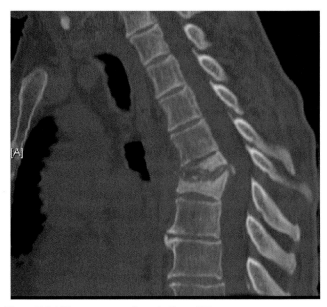

Figure 7.4 MRI appearances of case in Figure 7.3.

The mainstay of treatment is appropriate antibiotics, the duration of which is governed by the patient's general condition and the inflammatory markers.

Collections such as epidural abscesses may require draining.

An epidural abscess can present with an acute deterioration of the patient's neurology along with systemic upset. The ESR and white cell count (WCC) are almost always raised in these cases and an MRI confirms the diagnosis. The epidural abscess represents a surgical emergency, especially when associated with neurological deterioration.

Inflammatory arthropathy

Rheumatoid arthritis

Rheumatoid arthritis primarily affects the cervical spine but can also affect other regions of the spine. Ten percent of rheumatoid patients will present with cervical spondylitis as the initial manifestation. Cervical spine involvement occurs early in the disease process and causes reported neurological impairment in up to 58% of patients.

Occurring commonly in women in the age of 30 to 50, cervical instability is the most serious and potentially life-threatening manifestation of this disease.

Presentation

Neck pain and neurological symptoms are the main presenting complaints in rheumatoid disease of the spine. Up to 80% of rheumatoid patients may have neck pain and up to 50% will have neurology.

The neck pain is often occipital and associated with headaches. Myelopathic symptoms such as early weakness and gait disturbances may be seen. Hand function may be impaired. Sensory changes and sphincter disturbances are usually seen late in the presentation.

Examination of the spine and full neurological examination should be performed. Any findings consistent with myelopathy should prompt further investigations.

Investigations

Standard cervical X-rays must be obtained in the evaluation of the rheumatoid patient, including flexion and extension views.

MRI and CT scans are required in patients with either a neurological deficit or radiographic evidence of instability. MRI in addition will give information of the soft tissues and compression of the neural elements if present. CT scans will help in pre-operative planning.

Treatment

The goals of treatment are to prevent neurological injury, sudden death, reducing pain and restoring function. Many patients with radiographic changes will still be asymptomatic. In these patients, along with the medical control of their disease, supportive measures are all that are needed, which includes physiotherapy and occasionally cervical orthosis for pain relief. Annual radiographic follow-up is also required to detect instability and treat it before neurology develops. The indications for surgery are neurological impairment, instability and pain.

Ankylosing spondylitis

Ankylosing spondylitis is an inflammatory spondyloarthropathy that affects the spine and sacroiliac joints. Men are affected four times more than women. There is a strong association with human leukocyte antigen (HLA)-B27.

Presentation

The patient may present early with arthritic pain of the sacroiliac joints.

Morning stiffness can be the presenting problem. The spinal movements may be limited. As the spondylitis progresses, kyphosis can develop. The spondylitis normally progresses from caudal to cranial. Once the spine is ankylosed, the symptoms of pain resolve.

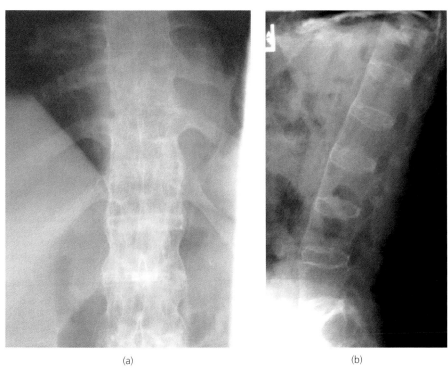

(a)   (b)

Figure 7.5 (a) X-ray appearances of ankylosing spondylitis. (b) X-ray appearances of ankylosing spondylitis.

Investigations

HLA-B27 can be positive in up to 96% of cases.

Radiographic findings include fusion of the sacroiliac joints. The annulus fibrosis ossifies sparing the anterior longitudinal ligament and the disc, giving rise to the 'bamboo spine' (Figure 7.5(a), (b)).

Treatment

Treatment is directed towards maintaining spinal alignment with exercises and stretching of the hip flexors and hamstrings for flexibility.

Spinal fractures in patients of Ankylosing spondilitis are easily missed. There should always be a high index of suspicion of a fracture even in a minor incident of trauma. There should be a low threshold for CT scanning such patients after appropriate immobilization.

Others

Other inflammatory arthropathies such as psoriases, Reiter's syndrome, enteropathic spondyloarthropathy and diffuse idiopathic skeletal hyperostosis (DISH) can affect the spine. The symptoms are axial pain and stiffness similar to ankylosing spondylitis. DISH is another condition where there should be a low threshold for CT scanning the spine after trauma.

Further reading

Govender S. Spinal infections. *Journal of Bone and Joint Surgery* 2005; **87**(11): 1454–1458.

Patchell RA, Tibbs PA, Regine WF, *et al.* Direct decompressive surgical resection in the treatment of spinal cord compression caused by metastatic cancer: a randomised trial. *Lancet* 2005; **366**(9486): 643–648.

CHAPTER 8

Whiplash

Kate Prince[1], Andrew Clarke[2] and Alwyn Jones[3]

[1]General Practitioner, VTS Wessex, UK
[2]Royal Devon and Exeter Hospital, Devon, UK
[3]University Hospital of Wales, Cardiff, UK

OVERVIEW

- Whiplash associated disorders are very common and the frequency is increasing

- There is no succinct definition of this condition

- No consistent tissue injury has been identified

- A thorough history and examination is essential at the initial point of contact

- Reassurance, advice and early active intervention are the best approach

---

The history of whiplash

Crowe is credited with coining the term 'whiplash' in 1928 during a symposium. However, whiplash first entered the world literature in 1945, when Davis described it as hyperflexion followed by spontaneous recoil. Gay and Abbott added to the growing writings, noting rear impacts as a major cause.

Yet, in 1955 Severy studied the mechanism of whiplash on humans and dummies, concluding that there was a hyperextension followed by a flexion. So, within 10 years, the mechanism was turned on its head. Subsequent work by McConnell in 1995 found the first movement to be head rotation, followed by forward translation of the entire head, hence muddying the waters further.

Crowe, in 1963, felt that he had created a monster, and was quoted as saying he had used an unfortunate term. The expression was intended to be a description of motion, but it has been accepted by physicians, patients and lawyers as the name of a disease.

In 1995, the Quebec Task Force suggested using 'whiplash associated disorders' (WAD), as a catchall, because the symptoms that patients complained about were not only confined to the neck.

Definition

As there appears to be a constellation of symptoms associated with mechanisms of injury that provoke a 'whiplash associated disorder',

there currently is no succinct statement that describes it. Hence, we feel that it should be defined as a syndrome, with a common causal factor but a host of different manifestations, some of which are physical, others psychological and some fiduciary. Furthermore, it needs to be sub-divided into acute and chronic, as the approach to the patients will be different.

The Quebec Task Force definition states that whiplash is an acceleration–deceleration mechanism of energy transferred to the neck. However, they then describe the causes and consequences of such an event. Thus a very broad definition ensues. Other authors have narrowed the field to exclude any bony injury.

Epidemiology

In the United Kingdom 1 in 200 people have a WAD every year. This costs the United Kingdom £3 billion in litigation. In the United States, in 1996, there were more than 13 million motor vehicle accidents, of which 1 million resulted in WADs. The cost was estimated at $29 billion. However, in Lithuania, there were no reported incidences of chronic whiplash, despite some enthusiastic driving during a prospective controlled inception cohort study. Forty-seven percent of patients had initial symptoms, but by 1 year, they had no more symptoms than a matched cohort who had not been involved in a rear end collision.

Aetiology

The common causal factor is a road traffic accident. A rear impact is twice as likely to result in a whiplash type injury. Other activities can provoke such an injury, where there is a rapid acceleration and deceleration of the head relative to the body, such as contact sports.

Melville wrote to the Canadian Medical Association Journal in 1963, having witnessed demolition derbies. Despite observing 'heads flailing through a great range of motion' following high speed collisions, including rear impacts, there were no reported injuries.

Clinical features

Symptoms

Neck pain occurs in 62 to 100% and is the index symptom. This neck pain can radiate up, into the occipital region, across the

ABC of Spinal Disorders. Edited by Andrew Clarke, Alwyn Jones, Michael O'Malley and Robert McLaren.
© 2010 by Blackwell Publishing, ISBN: 978-1-4051-7069-7.

Table 8.1 Symptoms.

Symptoms of whiplash
Neck pain
Shoulder pain
Arm pain
Headache
Tinnitus
Visual symptoms
Dizziness
Low back pain
Temporomandibular joint symptoms
Paraesthesia
Concentration and memory Disturbance

shoulder and into the mid-scapular region. The neck pain can be posterior or anterior, usually located within the muscle bulk of trapezius posteriorly and of sternocleidomastoid anteriorly. Headaches, especially in the sub-occipital region are reported by up to 82% of patients (Table 8.1).

Associated ailments reported by patients include paraethesiae of the upper limb in almost 50%, and thoracolumbar back pain in 50%. Additional reports describe dysphagia, vertigo, audiovisual disturbances and cognitive impairment.

Signs

There are no pathognomonic physical signs associated with WAD. Almost 20% of patients will be found to have altered neurology, mostly in the upper limbs. These can be sensory or motor and even reduced reflexes.

Management

The management of WAD patients is divided conveniently into acute and chronic. With the acute injury, there is a window of opportunity to avoid the chronic stage, which drains both patient and practitioner. Some studies suggest up to a quarter of patients take more than 6 months to return to pre-injury levels of activity. Worse still, almost 10% develop some form of permanent disability.

A recent paper by Lankester *et al.* 2006 sought to identify factors predicting outcome after whiplash in patients involved in litigation. While this may well represent a massive bias towards chronicity and the display of illness behaviour, they found that the strongest factors were present prior to the injury (Table 8.2).

Additional factors cited are severity of acute symptoms, duration of symptoms, advancing age, gender, occipital headache and neurological signs.

Table 8.2 Risks of chronicity.

Physical	Psychological
Pre-injury back pain	Pre-injury depression or anxiety symptoms
Front position in vehicle	–
Pain radiating away from neck after injury	–

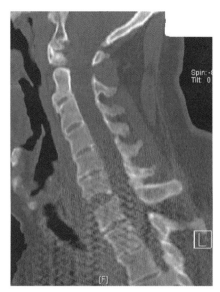

Figure 8.1 Mid-sagittal CT scan of cervical spine, with fracture through C6-7 disc space in patient with ankylosing spondylitis.

Acute management

Serious injuries must be ruled out at this stage. A detailed history is required, especially asking about conditions that make the neck vulnerable to significant instability with minimal trauma, for example, ankylosing spondylitis (Figure 8.1). Failure to do so could have terminal consequences for the patient.

A thorough clinical examination is mandatory. This should include a full neurological assessment. Imaging is not routinely required, as it is rarely helpful. However, the Canadian Cervical Spine X-ray guidelines can be used to help decide if plain radiographs are appropriate.

Once the clinical assessment has been performed, a concise and informative description of the problem should be discussed with the patient. The actual treatment following that discussion is the source of ongoing debate.

Historically, the advice was to use rest, analgesia and muscle relaxants. Often, immobilization with a soft collar for 2 to 4 weeks has also been employed.

Unsurprisingly, there is much debate as to the best way to manage these patients, in order to achieve the best recovery. There have been a multitude of prospective randomized controlled trials assessing the use of active intervention with therapists. Mealy *et al.* (1986) found patients had better outcomes with physical therapy. McKinney (1989) reported no difference if patients were given a home-based self-administered programme or an outpatient physical therapy programme. However, both groups were better than the third group who underwent a period of rest.

A further trial by Borchgrevink *et al.* (1999) described better recovery for patients advised to 'act as normal' versus patients given collars and rest. The patients who continued as normal had a better outcome at 6 months.

The question of cost has been raised for active intervention protocols. A recently reported study by Rosenfeld *et al.* (2006) suggested that active management with early exercises was cost-effective when compared to an information leaflet and advice.

The latest Cochrane review in 2006 found a trend for active interventions over passive ones. Yet, no firm conclusions were drawn on the basis of the available evidence.

Chronic management

Chronic whiplash syndrome can be defined as symptoms persisting beyond 6 months. It is characterized by a similar constellation of symptoms seen in the acute setting. However, there is a suspicion by some that the involvement of litigation by this time coupled with long-term disability makes management very challenging.

No study has so far identified a consistent tissue abnormality. Some authors have discussed chronic whiplash in terms of a functional somatic syndrome. Therefore, their therapy is targeted at that.

With this in mind, a six-step management plan can be implemented along the lines of Barsk and Borus's recommendations (Table 8.3).

Vendrig, Van Akkerveeken and McWhorter reported that a multi-modal treatment programme, including cognitive behavioural therapy for chronic whiplash, had resulted in 65% of patients returning to normal by 6 months and only 19% had sought further medical consultation for ongoing symptoms.

Whiplash and litigation

Compensation is often cited as a motivating factor for patients complaining of whiplash. Bellamy (1997) remarked that despite our best intentions to compensate those injured either by others' negligence or in the line of duty, we have perpetrated widespread iatrogenic illness.

It has been observed that return to work after occupational injuries is slower than for leisure injuries. After all, you have been injured by someone else. Apportioning blame and recognition of suffering are intricately woven into this condition.

However, viewing the literature as a whole, there is a consistency in the clinical picture, and few differences in outcomes between those claiming compensation versus those not claiming. Symptoms do improve with active management, even in patients involved in litigation, and the payment of compensation is not marked with an improved clinical picture.

Prognosis

This is often the question posed to practitioners. Bannister and Gargan reported in 1993 that the final outcome is determined by 2 years and probably much earlier. Approximately 70% of patients have reached their endpoint by 1 year. The literature suggests that about 50% of patients make a full recovery and up to 10% become chronically disabled. Almost 40% of those injured will either take time off work or become unemployed as a result of the injury.

However, the reported figures in the literature vary according to the population being studied and the insurance/compensation system that is pertinent to them.

Conclusions

Whiplash is a controversial subject. The history of whiplash charts rise from a description of a mechanism of injury to the status of an industry.

Logan and Holt (2003) concluded that staff with greater experience made more appropriate decisions, which included advice on exercise, utilization of physiotherapy and the absence of soft collars. This represents a key aspect in the management of acute whiplash and hopefully the avoidance of chronic whiplash.

Further reading

Bellamy R. Editorial comment. *Clinical Orthopaedics and Related Research* 1997; **336**: 2–3.

Cote P, Cassidy JD, Carroll L *et al.* A systematic review of the prognosis of acute whiplash and a new conceptual framework to synthesize the literature. *Spine* 2001; **26**(19): E445–E458.

Livingstone M. Whiplash injury: why are we achieving so little? *Journal of the Royal Society of Medicine* 2000; **93**: 526–529.

Mayou R, Radanov BP. Whiplash neck injury *Journal of Psychosomatic Research* 1996; **40**(5): 461–474.

Verhagen AP, Scholten-Peeters GGM, de Bie RA *et al.* Conservative treatments for whiplash. *The Cochrane Database of Systematic Reviews* 2006; (4): Art No. CD003338.

Waddell G, Burton K, McClune T. *The Whiplash Book.* The Stationery Office, London, 2001.

Young WF. The enigma of whiplash. *Postgraduate Medicine* 2001; **109**(3). 179–186.

References

Borchgrevink GE, Kassa A, McDonagh D *et al.* Acute treatment of whiplash neck strain injuries: a randomised controlled trial of treatment during the first 14 days after a car accident. *Spine* 1998; **23**: 25–31.

Lankester BJA, Garneti N, Gargan MF. *et al.* Factors predicting the outcome of whiplash injury in subjects pursuing litigation. *European Spine Journal* 2006; **15**: 902–907.

Logan AJ, Holt MD. Management of whiplash injuries presenting to accidnet and emergency departments in Wales. *Emergency Medical Journal* 2003; **20**: 354–355.

McKinney LA. The role of physiotherapy in the management of acute neck sprains following road traffic accidents. *Archives of Emergency Medicine* 1989; **6**: 27–33.

Mealy K, Brennan H, Fenelou GC. Early mobilisation of acute whiplash injuries. *British Medical Journal (Clinical research Ed)* 1986; **292**: 656–657.

Rosenfeld M, Seferiadis A, Gunnarsson R. Active involvement and intervention in patients exposed to whiplash trauma in automobile crashes reduces costs. A randomised controlled trial and health economic evaluation. *Spine* 2006; **31**(16): 1799–1804.

Table 8.3 Management plan.

Step	Strategy
One	Exclude treatable causes
Two	Search for psychiatric disorders
Three	Form partnership with patient
Four	Set functional restoration as goal
Five	Provide reassurance
Six	Use cognitive behavioural therapy for resistant cases

CHAPTER 9

Osteoporosis and Osteoporotic Spinal Fractures

John R. Andrews

Consultant Spinal Surgeon, Newcastle, UK

OVERVIEW

- Osteoporosis is a very common problem, causing much morbidity
- Approximately 1 in 3 women and 1 in 12 males older than 50 have osteoporosis
- There are no specific symptoms, until a fracture occurs
- Some risk factors are modifiable to reduce risks of fracture
- Diagnosis requires a DEXA scan
- Causes such as myeloma need ruling out in patients with wedge fractures

---

Osteoporosis

Introduction

Osteoporosis can be described as changes occurring in bones that cause decreased bone strength and an increased risk of fracture. Bone is a living structure that, when healthy, undergoes a constant balanced destruction and production by osteoclasts and osteoblasts respectively. Osteoporosis involves a loss of this balance, resulting in destruction occurring faster than regeneration. This in turn causes a reduced bone mass and disruption of the normal micro-architecture of bone. The World Health Organization's definition of osteoporosis is a bone mineral density (BMD) of 2.5 or more standard deviations (SDs) below normal peak bone mass (T score <-2.5).

Osteoporosis is commoner with increasing age. Peak bone mass is obtained at the approximate age of 30; it then plateaus for a 10-year period. After approximately 40 years of age, an age-related decline in bone mass starts. Oestrogen has a significant effect on age-related bone loss in women and men. Vitamin D deficiency and secondary hyperparathyroidism are common in the elderly population and may contribute. Decreased activity levels and a decrease in insulin-like growth factors have also been postulated to be important.

Peak bone mass is an important factor in osteoporosis as subsequent age-related bone loss will have a greater effect on those individuals starting with a low peak bone mass. Peak bone mass is less in women than men, and genetic factors are another major determinant of peak bone density. Nutrition, especially calcium and vitamin D intake, hormonal status and degree of physical activity have all been shown to affect peak bone mass.

Osteoporosis risk factors

- **Sex** – women are more affected than men; this is due to a lower starting peak bone mass, increased bone loss at the menopause and a greater life expectancy.
- Age.
- Previous fragility fracture.
- Family history of osteoporosis and maternal history of hip fracture.
- Early menopause.
- Steroid treatment.
- Other drugs (aromatase inhibitors, androgen deprivation therapy).
- Smoking.
- Alcohol intake (>3 units per day).
- Body mass index <19.

Some diseases are associated with osteoporosis including the following:

- Rheumatoid arthritis
- Untreated hypogonadism
- Malabsorption
- Endocrine disease
- Chronic liver disease
- Chronic renal disease
- Chronic obstructive airway disease.

Clinical presentation

Osteoporotic fracture is the commonest clinical presentation of osteoporosis (Figure 9.1). A low-energy fall (from a standing height or less) causing a fracture should raise suspicion of osteoporosis in an adult. However, in spinal osteoporotic fractures, as many as one-third of patients who suffer a fracture are asymptomatic. These

---

ABC of Spinal Disorders. Edited by Andrew Clarke, Alwyn Jones, Michael O'Malley and Robert McLaren.
© 2010 by Blackwell Publishing, ISBN: 978-1-4051-7069-7.

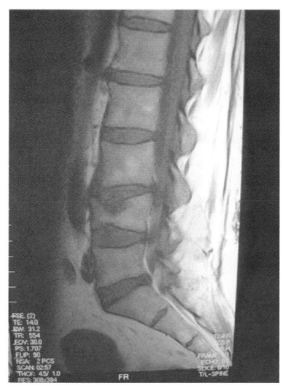

Figure 9.1 Osteoporotic fracture demonstrated on MRI.

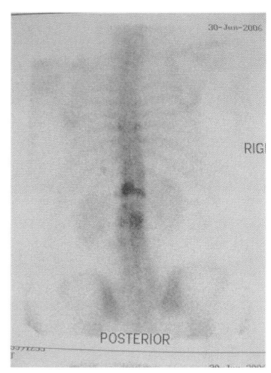

Figure 9.2 Bone scan showing osteoporotic fractures in patient with no history of trauma.

cases may later present with back pain, a decrease in height or spinal deformity (Figure 9.2). Osteoporosis can also be diagnosed from the screening of at-risk populations.

Investigations

Techniques to diagnose osteoporosis on plain radiography are very subjective and their reliability has been shown to be poor. The gold standard is dual energy X-ray absorptiometry (DEXA). Results are given as a T score, which is a value of the SD of BMD from normal peak bone mass. It can also be given as a Z score which is the SD of BMD from age-matched controls. The World Health Organization definition is based on T values taken from the spine and hip. Other methods of diagnosis include quantitative computed tomography (CT) and ultrasound (usually of the calcaneum).

People who have suffered a previous fragility fracture are greatly at risk of another fracture and are labelled as having established osteoporosis if their T score is <−2.5. In older patients (National Institute for Clinical Excellence (NICE) advises older than 75) after a fracture, the diagnosis of osteoporosis is so likely that bone density measurements are not always necessary.

Although the World Health Organization's definition of osteoporosis indicates a significantly increased risk of fracture it is not uncommon for fragility-type fractures to occur below this defined level of BMD. Clinical risk factors should be borne in mind and tertiary referral may be appropriate as it can be beneficial to treat some patients with a BMD <2.5 SD below normal.

The following blood tests are advised in order to screen for secondary osteoporosis:

- Full blood count (FBC) plus erythrocyte sedimentation rate (ESR)
- Liver function tests
- Renal function tests
- Bone profile which includes calcium, phosphate and alkaline phosphatase
- Myeloma screen
- Thyroid function tests.

Treatment

Simple methods would involve the cessation of smoking and alcohol abuse with an increase in exercise/activity levels while ensuring an adequate diet. Vitamin D and calcium intake are essential components of diet, and supplements may be necessary.

Pharmacological treatment of osteoporosis should be started early as it is aimed at preventing future fractures and mortality, morbidity and disability associated with these fractures. NICE has given some prescribing guidance, which is available on its website. It is important to individualize treatments as not all drugs have been proved to be beneficial for all types of fractures and side effects, and drug interactions need to be considered. The majority of patients can be treated in primary care but younger patients, those who fail to respond to treatment or patients requiring intravenous (IV) or anabolic treatments are likely to benefit from tertiary input.

It is important to understand that while treating glucocorticoid-induced osteoporosis, the main effect of steroids on bone loss occurs during the first 6 to 12 months. Prophylactic treatment should, therefore, be started early in a patient who will be taking the equivalent of 7.5 mg prednisolone for more than 3 months.

Drugs available to treat osteoporosis include the following:

- Bisphosphonates are inhibitors of bone resorption and increase BMD by altering osteoclast activation and function. They are considered first-line treatments for post-menopausal osteoporosis. Complex administration protocols are a problem for compliance. The main side effect is gastrointestinal (GI) irritation. It is known that 20 to 30% of patients taking bisphosphonates stop their treatment within 12 months and 12 to 18% of patients report non-compliance, with at least one administration guideline. Monitoring is therefore very important.
- Strontium ranelate is thought to have a dual effect on bone metabolism, increasing bone formation and decreasing bone resorption. It is an alternative front-line treatment. Main side effects are mild including headache and diarrhoea.
- Of selective oestrogen receptor modulators (SERMs), the only drug currently licensed for use in osteoporosis raloxifene. It enhances the beneficial effects of oestrogen on bone. Second-line treatment is often used in younger women. Side effects include hot flushes, cramps and a three-time increase in venous thromboembolism. It is protective against breast cancer.
- Teraparatide is a recombinant, a fragment of human parathyroid hormone and being an anabolic agent, it stimulates new bone formation and increases resistance to fracture. Second line treatment is not proven against hip fracture. The only mode of delivery is by subcutaneous injection and it is expensive.
- Hormone replacement therapy is generally a second-line option. This therapy is most suitable for young post-menopausal women.
- Calcium and vitamin D are not proven to be of benefit alone, except in institutionalized elderly people. The use of these two supplements is recommended in treatment of osteoporosis with other drugs as the trials on such drugs included these two supplements.

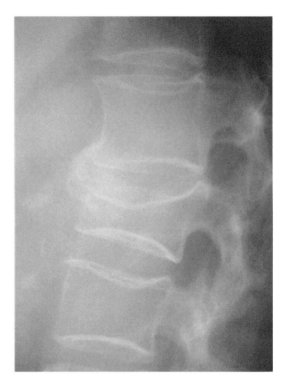

Figure 9.3 Pre-op X-ray of an osteoporotic fracture.

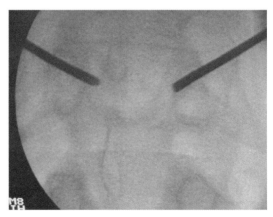

Figure 9.4 Anteroposterior (AP) X-ray demonstrating needle placement.

Osteoporotic fractures

Fractures caused by osteoporosis have been diagnosed in one in five men and one in two women older than 50. They are a major cause of morbidity and disability, resulting in an enormous cost to health service providers.

Treatment

The vast majority of osteoporotic spinal fractures can be successfully treated conservatively. Analgesia reduction in activity and bracing are the standard conservative methods used. Underlying osteoporosis should be treated to decrease the risk of further fractures.

In a small percentage of patients, conservative treatment fails and these patients can be considered for the following more invasive treatments.

Vertebroplasty

Vertebroplasty is the injection of acrylic bone cement into the vertebral body in order to relieve pain or stabilize the fractured vertebrae. It is performed under local or general anesthesia, generally using percutaneous needle techniques guided by fluoroscopy. The X-rays shown here are pre-operative (Figure 9.3), needle placement (Figures 9.4 and 9.5) and post-operative (Figure 9.6). The literature indicates some level of pain relief in 58 to 97% of patients, with an associated reduction in pain medication usage in 50 to 91% of patients. One study indicated that 93% of patients had improved mobility and that 100% of patients were satisfied with the procedure and would have it again. Multiple levels can be treated (Figure 9.7). It has been approved by NICE. Complications include neurological deterioration from incorrect catheter placement or cement leakage. Cement leakage has been reported in 25% of cases but only 1% of these leakages are said to clinically affect the patient. Cement embolism and subsequent pulmonary problems are also a concern.

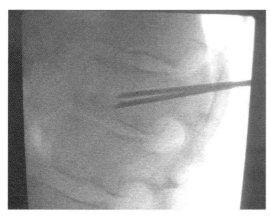

Figure 9.5 Lateral X-ray demonstrating needle placement.

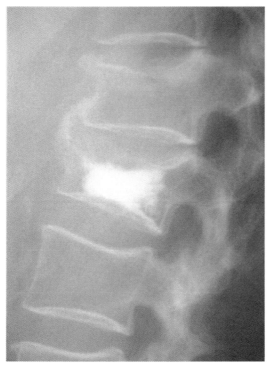

Figure 9.6 Post-operative X-ray appearance.

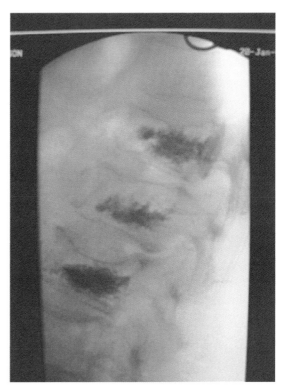

Figure 9.7 Multiple levels treated.

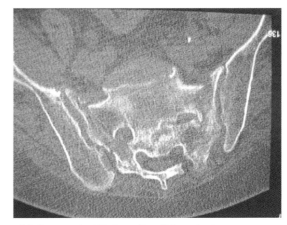

Figure 9.8 Pre-operative CT of sacral insufficiency fracture.

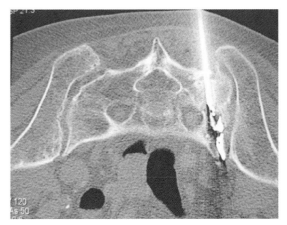

Figure 9.9 Needle placement and injection using CT guidance.

Sacroplasty

Sacral insufficiency fractures are particularly difficult to treat. Conservative treatment often involves a prolonged period of pain and suffering. Like vertebroplasty, bone cement is injected into the sacrum but CT guidance is useful in this area. The CTs shown are pre-operative (Figure 9.8), needle placement (Figure 9.9) and post-operative (Figure 9.10) pictures. Immediate decreases in pain scores are reported, with further improvements over the next weeks.

Kyphoplasty

This technique is similar to vertebroplasty but a balloon-like device (inflatable bone tamp) is inserted into the vertebral body. The balloon is slowly inflated under fluoroscopy until the normal height of the vertebral body is restored or the balloon reaches its

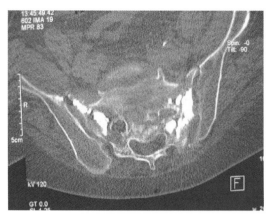

Figure 9.10 Post-operative CT image.

maximum volume. The balloon is then deflated, and the cavity created is filled with cement at a low pressure. The injection of cement at low pressure into the ready-made defect decreases but does not eliminate cement leakage.

Kyphoplasty enthusiasts state that the decrease in cement leakage, along with the increases in vertebral height and decreases in the degree of kyphosis gained by the use of the balloon, make it a better procedure than vertebroplasty. However, in studies to date, there is little evidence that the increased cost of the procedure and the rare balloon-related complications are justified by a significant change in the clinical patient outcome measures.

Surgery

Surgery in the presence of significant osteoporosis represents a major challenge. The use of larger diameter screws and bone cement will increase screw pull-out strengths and supplementary hooks and wires can spread the loads, making surgery possible. However, instrument failure is common and because of the elderly population involved the overall complication rate is very high. Reported complication rates for deformity surgery in the elderly are 50 to 70%. However, in these studies more than 70% of patients reported significant improvement and satisfaction with the procedures. Surgery should be reserved for cases with neurological deficit, major deformity or when other methods have already been exhausted.

Acknowledgements

I would like to thank my colleague Dr. Steven James (Consultant radiologist) for the images he allowed me to use to illustrate this chapter. These are taken from his own series of interventional radiology procedures performed on osteoporotic fractures.

Further reading

Cooper C, Atkinson EJ, O'Fallon WM *et al.* Incidence of clinically diagnosed vertebral fractures: a population based study in Rochester, Minnesota, 1985–1989. *Journal of Bone and Mineral Research* 1992; **7**: 221–227.

Cummings SR, Melton LJ. Epidemiology and outcomes of osteoporotic fractures. *Lancet* 2002; **359**: 1761–1767.

De Negri P, Tirri T, Paternoster G *et al.* Treatment of painful osteoporotic or traumatic vertebral compression fractures by percutaneous vertebral augmentation procedures: a nonrandomized comparison between vertebroplasty and kyphoplasty. *Clinical Journal of Pain* 2007; **23**(5): 425–430.

Frey M, DePalma M, Cifu D *et al.* Efficacy and safety of percutaneous sacroplasty for painful osteoporotic sacral insufficiency fractures: a prospective trial. *Spine* 2007; **32**(15): 1635–1640.

Guidelines working group for the bone and tooth society, and Royal College of Physicians. *Glucocorticoid Induced Osteoporosis: Guidelines for Prevention and Treatment.* Royal College of Physicians, London, 2002.

NICE guidelines on vertebroplasty and kyphoplasty. Balloon kyphoplasty for vertebral compression fractures. April 2006.

NICE published guidelines on osteoporosis diagnosis and treatment. Balloon kyphoplasty for vertebral compression fractures. April 2006.

Papaioannou, Alexandra, Kennedy, Courtney Dolovich *et al.* Patient adherence to osteoporosis medications: problems, consequences and management strategies. *Drugs & Aging* 2007; **24**(1): 37–55.

Poole K, Compston J. Osteoporosis and its management. *BMJ* 2006; **333**: 1251–1256.

CHAPTER 10

Physiotherapy in Spinal Conditions

Adrian Brown

Physiotherapist, Wales, UK

OVERVIEW

- Outline of physiotherapy
- Relevant referral
- Physiotherapy assessment and clinical reasoning
- Treatment types and their objectives

Physiotherapy

The objective of physiotherapy intervention in spinal management is to provide the client with a structured relevant process. This entails accurate assessment, clinical reasoning, data processing and diagnosis. This allows for the prescription of a treatment programme that provides the correct and relevant management for the client and his/her condition.

Physiotherapy provides optimal spinal function to an individual taking into consideration pathologies that may be present.

For normal spinal function to occur, all elements such as osseous, neural, muscular and soft tissue, must perform their individual roles and integrate with each other to maintain spinal homeostasis.

Damage or dysfunction to any of the above will have implications throughout the associated systems.

It is not only the physiotherapist's role to understand how each of these systems operates within a normal healthy system, but also to understand how and what effect alterations in one system will have on its associated reliant systems.

These changes may be due to trauma, pathology and altered biomechanical stresses, and may occur from any incident, accident or alterations that may have occurred at any time.

The physiotherapist must therefore build up a vast clinical knowledge to help, evaluate and manage the client's condition including background knowledge on socio-economic, psychosocial and the roles of the other health-care professionals within the spinal management team.

This clinical knowledge allows the physiotherapist to assess, evaluate, reason, diagnose, treat and provide a relevant management programme to achieve optimal spinal function. This is illustrated with an example as shown in Figure 10.1.

From the above example, it can be seen how alteration in one area can affect the normal inter-linking between the systems. For example, an acute disc injury such as a disc herniation sustained in loaded flexion and rotation, is likely to cause an increase in muscle tone. This limits stresses on the acutely inflamed disc, thereby limiting range of movement segmentally within the articular and neurodynamics systems.

These changes will alter the client's movement patterns causing altered stresses on other structures and possibly subjecting them to subsequent injury. (This client may present with the classic shifted S-shaped spine.)

In this example, if the physiotherapist is the initial contact, the assessment process would be used to diagnose and establish a management programme.

If, from this process the diagnosis of acute disc injury is established the client may present with the following problems.

1 Shifted S-shaped spine due to active increase in muscle tone (in large global muscles).
2 Segmental decrease in range of movement at effected level (joint held in locked position).
3 Limited neurodynamics (limited straight-legged raise or slump tests).
4 Inhibition of functional control/stability in muscles (small segmental muscles such as tranverse abdominal and multifidus).
5 Alteration to all functional movement patterns.

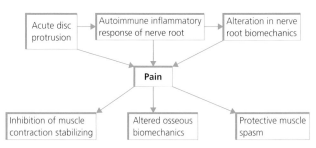

Figure 10.1 Illustration of interaction between systems using disc prolapse as an example.

ABC of Spinal Disorders. Edited by Andrew Clarke, Alwyn Jones, Michael O'Malley and Robert McLaren.
© 2010 by Blackwell Publishing, ISBN: 978-1-4051-7069-7.

The physiotherapist has to decide a management strategy that will benefit the client. From clinical experience an expected time-period and patient education can be provided.

The physiotherapist has to decide which element of the inter-linked system to prioritize; this may well be selected on clinical response during assessment or clinical experience.

The alternate treatment strategies as shown in Figure 10.1 are as follows:

1 Manual therapy at the affected joint returning normal joint biomechanics, joint movement and function.
   Providing decrease in pain and global muscle spasm.
   Improvement in neurodynamics and stabilizing muscle recruitment.
   Thereby, allowing the client to return to his/her normal posture and movement patterns.
2 Alternatively the therapist may decide to treat the global muscle increase and release of this may provide the same result as above.

Criteria for physiotherapy referral

Certain criteria are required for physiotherapy to be effective and beneficial to the client. Figure 10.2 provides a quick reference to effective referral.

Physiotherapists are often used as a triage service where they are the initial contact.

From their assessment and clinical knowledge, the most effective management strategy for the client can be established (as shown in Figure 10.2).

It can be seen that a competent initial triage can provide the client with an effective management pathway relevant to his/her condition and initial assessment by a competent physiotherapist is probably the most effective way of establishing that pathway. This allows the therapist to establish the problem, treat and/or refer on as appropriate.

This management strategy may include liaison with other members of the management team such as follows:

1 Consultants' constant communication between the spinal consultant and the spinal physiotherapist is required as the therapist spends a greater period of time with the client and often the rapport allows for further relevant information to be collected.
2 General practitioners – Often the referring party keep them informed, discuss treatment and provide discharge data, which helps them reinforce the management provided.
3 Physiotherapy peers.
4 Radiological personnel – Further ongoing investigations and investigation reports are often discussed and interventions such as nerve root blocks and facet joint injections are often used to aid the therapist with their treatment plan.
5 Pain management clinics – Management of chronic back conditions is often a complex team effort co-ordinated by a lead therapist.
6 Other relevant persons such as carers, coaches and employers.

It can be seen that quite often the physiotherapist is the one person spending more quality time with the client assessing treatment and will often be the individual pulling all the relevant persons, results and information together.

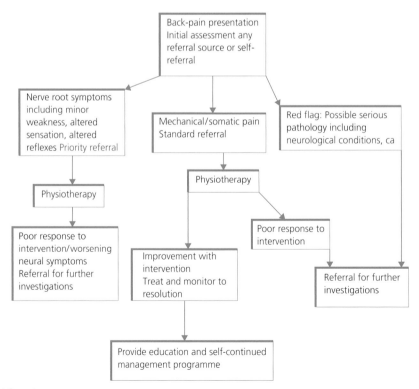

Figure 10.2 Relevant referral flow chart.

Physiotherapy management clinical reasoning process

Step 1: Subjective assessment

Subjective assessment at this stage should cover all aspects of the problem as related by the client, and must include the following:

Problem
- Type/nature, pain, dysfunction stiffness
- aggravating/easing factors
- Irritability (aggravating and settling times)
- Duration
- History
- Onset (gradual, aggressive)
- Possible causes (incidents, changes to routine or life style)
- Progression or regression.

Past medical history including previous episodes or injuries
Drug history

Social circumstances, work type, leisure activities and changes in life style.

The above information will allow the clinician to form a detailed picture of the client and his/her problem. Using clinical experience and a clinical reasoning thought process a working theory can be established. This provides the basis for the selection of objective tests that are relevant to confirm or negate the working theory/diagnosis. (You cannot test everything on all clients.)

Subjective information, investigations and objective physical examination are all analyzed to establish the working theory/diagnosis. This, then, provides a working theory that allows a management plan to be established, which provides short- and long-term management goals (as shown in Figure 10.3).

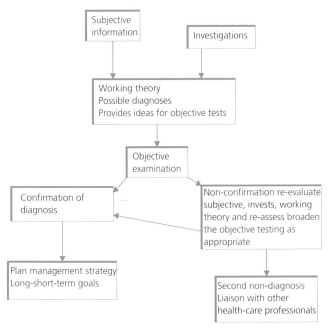

Figure 10.3 Summary of clinical reasoning process.

Physiotherapy interventions

The physiotherapist, having established the problem/diagnosis and subsequent treatment goals, has a number of techniques that may be effective (Table 10.1), using one or a combination of techniques to achieve the treatment goals.

Manual techniques

The manual techniques tend to those techniques carried out by the physiotherapist.

1 Adjustments or joint manipulations used to restore joint range and release protective spasm.
2 Mulligan's techniques and joint gliding techniques aimed at restoring the natural joint biomechanics.

Passive

1 *Electrotherapy*: Electrical equipment, ultrasound, laser, interferential that is used to help limit inflammatory changes, reduce muscle spasm and promote healing.
2 *Ice/heat*: Used to decrease inflammatory changes and decrease muscle spasm.

Exercise intervention
Rehabilitation techniques

1 *Muscle flexibility and core stability*: It is essential that muscles function at the correct length, with sufficient strength and are recruited at the precise time of requirement. If any of these factors are deficient then normal efficient function cannot be performed.
2 All strengthening and cardiovascular training as long as it is appropriate to the client and their treatment goals is relevant.

Education

Probably, physiotherapy is the most powerful treatment technique available to the physiotherapist educating the client about his/her

Table 10.1 Sample of physiotherapy techniques.

Manual intervention	Passive	Exercise intervention	Education
Manual therapy/ manipulation	Electrotherapy	Muscle imbalance	Condition/ prognosis
Mulligans/ Kaltenbourne	Ice	Muscle flexibility	Causes/prevention
Muscle energy techniques	–	Core strengthening	Lifestyle changes
Soft tissue release	–	Pilates	Fitness/health in relevance to the condition
McKenzie	–	Gym work, strength CV, control and muscle recruitment and timing	–
Neural mobilizations	–	–	–

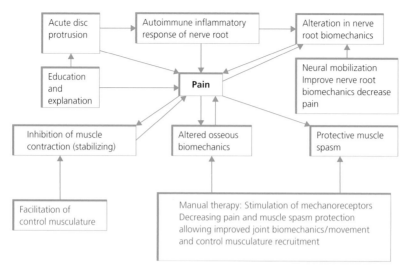

Figure 10.4 Illustration of intervention techniques using example as shown in Figure 10.1.

diagnosis right through his/her management including treatment options, lifestyle changes, ergonomics and exercise.

This education is provided to all persons associated with the client including carers, employers and family (Figure 10.4).

Possible intervention for above example

Manual therapy mobilization, manipulation aimed at restoring joint biomechanics thus decreasing protective spasm allowing easier recruitment, less inhibition of the stabilizing musculature and allowing normalization of neural biomechanics. All these factors produce an alteration in pain response, improved function and an early return to normality.

The physiotherapist will use a combination of the above skills during the various stages of the client's management depending on the condition and its prognosis. Most important is the education and information provided not only during treatment but after, to allow the client to manage and/or prevent further problems in the future.

Further reading

Bogduk Nikolai. Clinical Anatomy of the Lumbar Spine and Sacrum.

Fritz Julie N. Clinical reasoning strategies in physiotherapy.

McKenzie Robin. Treat your own back.

McKenzie Robin. Treat your own neck.

Richards Carolyn, Jull GA, Hides JA *et al*. Therapeutic exercise for spinal segmental stabilization in low back pain.

CHAPTER 11

Osteopathy

Walter Llewellyn McKone

Osteopath, London, UK

OVERVIEW

- Osteopathy considers the spine as one organ
- Musculoskeletal derangement and pathology is termed **somatic dysfunction**
- Somatic dysfunction is not central but inclusive in osteopathic diagnosis and treatment
- Somatic dysfunction is considered the end result of total patient–environment disturbance
- Diagnosis of somatic dysfunction considers evidence-based modalities of general medical practice and palpation of anatomically related tissues
- Treatment of somatic dysfunction considers evidenced-based surgical, pharmacologic, psychological, nutritional, manipulative and lifestyle interventions

---

'The object of this corporation is to establish a College of Osteopathy, the design of which is to improve our present system of surgery, obstetrics and treatment of diseases generally, and place the same on a more rational and scientific basis, and to impart information to the medical profession, and to grant and confer such honours and degrees as are usually granted and conferred by reputable medical colleges; to issue diplomas in testimony of the same to all students graduating from said school under the seal of the corporation, with the signature of each member of the faculty and the president of the college.'

– (Booth, 1924)

Placing the school on a 'rational and scientific basis' placed the thinking osteopaths with their judgement and reasoning at the centre of the healing system essentially turning osteopaths into

Introduction

Osteopathy was discovered by Andrew Taylor Still, MD (1828–1917) (Figure 11.1). He hailed from Kansas, USA, and was a practising physician during the mid-nineteenth and early twentieth century. He attended the College of Physicians and Surgeons in Kansas and served on the Kansas Free Assembly and State Legislator and worked formally for the abolition of slavery between 1857 and 1858. Having served in the American Civil War as a scout surgeon in the Ninth Kansas Cavalry, he returned home and within weeks witnessed the death of four of his children to spinal meningitis. It was the death of his children that drove him to reform, not pose an alternative to or complement the then practice of medicine. Returning to the study of anatomy and making it the central tenet of his study he announced the discovery of osteopathy in 1874. In 1892, Still established the American School of Osteopathy at Kirksville, Missouri, with the issuing of a new Charter in 1894 under the law regulating educational institutions. Article three, which clearly sets forth the purposes and powers of the school, is as follows:

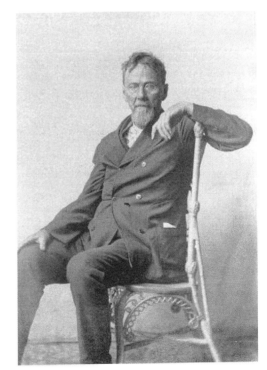

A. T. Still, c. 1903

Figure 11.1 Picture of Andrew Taylor Still.

ABC of Spinal Disorders. Edited by Andrew Clarke, Alwyn Jones, Michael O'Malley and Robert McLaren.
© 2010 by Blackwell Publishing, ISBN: 978-1-4051-7069-7.

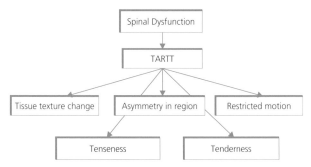

Figure 11.2 The mnemonic TARTT (**T**issue, **A**ssymetry, **R**estricted, **T**enseness and **T**enderness) in mechanical spinal dysfunction.

philosopher-physicians. 'My object is to make the osteopath a philosopher, and place him on the rock of reason. Then I will not have to worry of writing details of how to treat any organ of the human body, because he is qualified to the degree of knowing what has produced variations of all kinds in form and motion.' (Still, 1910) A modern approach to the original philosophy, principles and practice of osteopathy can be found in a more phenomenological approach to medicine (Baron, 1985 and McKone, 2001).

The spine

Any discussion of the spine as a stand-alone entity is osteopathically artificial. Spinal column anatomy, physiology and development are considered as early as embryonic somite and segment formation. The base of the spinal column from a developmental standpoint is considered to be the second to fourth thoracic segments. In standing position, the spinal column is more vulnerable as its function is reliant on the mobility of the hips and any significant length discrepancy of the lower limbs. Increased functional demand is placed on the cervico-thoracic and lumbo-sacral junctional regions because of a change in mobility from the mobile cervical segments to the relatively immobile thoracic segments and the mobile lumbar segments to the immobile sacrum.

For the osteopath, the spine is a multi-segmental single organ housing and protecting a significant portion of the central nervous system with the cumulative form of each vertebra providing ligament and muscle attachments for movement guided by the articular facets or apophyseal joints. Intervertebral discs provide the binding of vertebra-to-vertebra, somatosensory feedback and shock absorption. Collectively the skin, muscle, tendon and fascial complex is known as the **somatic component** (Figure 11.2).

Somatic dysfunction

A major contribution to the development of the somatic approach to spinal function and dysfunction was the kinematic analytical approach of Hoag, Kosok and Moser (1960). This quantitative approach developed into the somatic model to clearly define examination, diagnosis and manipulation of single and multi-segmental spinal levels (Johnston, 1988). Each vertebral segmental level has a corresponding spinal cord segmental level. Through the spinal cord segment visceral reflexes from heart, lungs, liver, bladder and so on, influence the somatic component leading to a viscero-somatic or somato-visceral reflex component, the direction of the stimulus depending on the origin of the stimulus towards the spinal cord (Figure 11.3). Alteration in reflex function from visceral, somatic or both sources can lead to corresponding alteration in tissue fluid content, arterio-venous circulation, lymphatic drainage and joint mobility. In addition, the disturbance of joint mobility affects the interface of the soft disc and hard vertebral bone with shock absorption and movement demands increasing the possibility of bulge and herniation of discs between levels C5 to C7-T1 and the L3 to L5-S1.

Pain is reciprocal with maintained nociceptive autonomic reflex activity, inflammation and changes in visceral and immunologic function leading to immediate functional and long-term pathologic changes (Van Buskirk, 1990). Nociceptive autonomic reflex activity is prevalent in the sympathetic portion of the autonomic nervous system leading to disruption in arterio-venous and lymphatic function (Elenkov, Wilder *et al.*, 2000). Single or multi-segmental spinal dysfunction can be purely mechanical, indicative of spinal pathology and/or a reflexive indicator of underlying visceral disease.

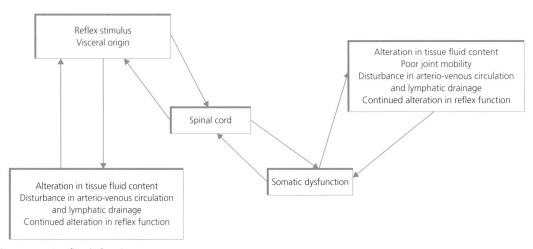

Figure 11.3 Viscero-somatic reflex dysfunction.

Single and multi-segmental spinal dysfunction and pathology results generally from the following:

- Age
- Infection
- Trauma
- Poor nutrition
- Lifestyle
- Occupation
- Psychological distress.

Single and multi-segmental spinal dysfunction and pathology results specifically from the following:

- Poor arterial-venous circulation
- Poor lymphatic circulation
- Altered vertebra-to-vertebra functional relationship
- Increasing muscular-ligament fibrosis
- Viscerosomatic aberrant reflexes.

Single or multi-segmental spinal dysfunction and pathology presents as follows:

- Pain
- Oedema
- Lymphadenopathy
- Joint limitation
- Guarding
- Soft tissue contracture or wasting
- Spasm
- Dryness of skin.

Single and multi-segmental dysfunction and pathology is indicative of some of the following spinal findings that are as follows:

- Occipital neuralgia
- Annulus fibrosis tear
- Disc protrusion and herniation
- Apophyseal joint inflammation
- Osteophytes
- General degeneration
- Ankylosing spondylitis
- Foraminal encroachment
- Radiculopathy
- Spasmodic torticollis.

Examination and diagnosis

An extensive system's case history is paramount followed by a general and specific examination. A general medical examination would involve cardiorespiratory, abdominal and neurological assessment. The specific assessment would follow any red flag indicative during the general assessment.

Spinal examination includes the following procedures:

Standing observation – posture, visceroptosis, contractures, scoliosis, and so on

Standing active movement ranges – flexion, extension and rotation

Sitting spinal assessment – active ranges and passive examination. Supine and prone passive examination.

During a passive examination the osteopath palpates and takes the segment or segments through a range of movements while the patient is relaxed. Depending on the texture of the soft tissues and the comfortable joint range and direction, the osteopath can assess the degree and extent of dysfunction. Any case history, examination or palpatory findings indicative of pathology are sent for further tests.

Intervention protocols

Depending on clinical findings intervention can take the following forms:

- Nutritional advice
- Pain control
- Exercises
- Psychotherapy
- Manipulation of restricted segments and soft tissue
- Referral to general medical practitioner.

Osteopathic manipulative medicine

This is the use of palpation followed by local or distant gentle stretching of soft tissues and passive joint movement. In most acute presentations local tissue is not touched and intervention is distant from the site of pain to reduce over-activity of the sympathetic nervous system presenting and influencing arousal and pain.

The aim of manipulation is to:

- Reduce aberrant reflex activity
- Improve arterio-venous circulation
- Improve lymphatic drainage
- Reduce oedema
- Reduce protective spasm
- Reduce visceral reflexes.

Further reading

Baron RJ. An introduction to medical phenomenology: I can't hear you while I'm listening. *Annuals of Internal Medicine* 1985; **103**: 606–611.

Booth ER. *History of Osteopathy and Twentieth-Century Medical Practice*. The Caxton Press, Cincinnati, Ohio, 1924.

Elenkov IJ, Wilder RL, Chrousos GP *et al*. The sympathetic nerve – an integrative interface between two supersystems: the brain and the immune system. *Pharmacological Review* 2000; **52**: 595–638.

Hoag JM, Kosok M, Moser JR. Kinematic analysis and classification of vertebral motion. *Journal of the American Osteopathic Association* 1960; **59**: 899–986.

Johnston WL. Segmental definition: Part 1. A focal point for diagnosis of somatic dysfunction. *Journal of the American Osteopathic Association* 1988; **88** (1): 99–105.

McKone WL. *Osteopathic Medicine: Philosophy, Principles and Practice*. Blackwell Science, Oxford, 2001.

Still AT. *Osteopathy – Research and Practice*. Kirksville, Missouri, 1910.

Van Buskirk RL. Nociceptive reflexes and the somatic dysfunction: a model. *Journal of the American Osteopathic Association* 1990; **90**(9): 792–809.

CHAPTER 12

Chiropractic

Richard Brown

Consultant Chiropractor, Gloucestershire, UK

OVERVIEW

- Chiropractors are highly trained back pain specialists
- Chiropractors offer a package of care, not just spinal manipulation
- Statutory regulation is by the General Chiropractic Council
- Evidence based treatment for acute and chronic spinal pain
- A safe intervention in the treatment of spinal disorders

Introduction

The modern practice of chiropractic in the United Kingdom has undergone a marked transformation over the last 20 years. Its progress can be largely attributed to the passing of the Chiropractors Act in 1994, heralding a milestone in the evolution of a profession that hitherto had been regarded with suspicion by the mainstream medical establishment. The rise of chiropractic popularity has also been due to an ever-increasing evidence base for both spinal manipulation and a biopsychosocial approach to the management of spinal disorders.

Now a mainstream health-care profession, chiropractic occupies an important position as one of the foremost specialist providers of non-surgical management of back pain. The inclusion of spinal manipulation in the Department of Health's Musculoskeletal Services Framework and within the NICE Guidelines for the treatment of chronic low back pain placed chiropractic at the heart of an innovative and multidisciplinary approach for managing a problem thought to cost the National Health Service (NHS) more than £1 billion annually.

Chiropractic is regulated in the United Kingdom by the General Chiropractic Council (GCC). The smallest of the statutory regulators, the GCC's primary remit is to protect patients, although it is also responsible for setting standards of conduct and practice. Such regulation means that GPs and consultants can now refer patients without being responsible for the chiropractor's actions and many chiropractors are now involved in providing care within local Primary Care Trust s (PCTs).

What is chiropractic?

Chiropractic is a health profession concerned with the diagnosis, treatment and prevention of mechanical disorders of the musculoskeletal system, particularly the spine, and the effects of these disorders on the function of the nervous system and on general health. Although chiropractors treat all joints, their particular expertise lies in dealing with back pain.

The main aim of chiropractic treatment is to restore normal function to the musculoskeletal system. By the careful assessment of joint function and general health through careful history taking, physical examination and, where appropriate, the use of diagnostic imaging, chiropractors are able to accurately identify and manage the majority of spinal disorders.

Modern chiropractic is not an alternative health profession but one which complements medical management by providing highly skilled, non-surgical treatment of common spinal disorders. Emphasis is placed on a comprehensive, biopsychosocial approach to management in line with current best evidence. While they are highly skilled in spinal manipulation, this is only one part of a package of care that also includes providing information, reassurance and advice, soft tissue techniques, exercise prescription, spinal rehabilitation programmes and ancillary techniques such as electrotherapy and myofascial dry needling.

Table 12.1 outlines appropriate referrals to a chiropractor.

Education and training

Chiropractic training in the United Kingdom has been provided at the degree level since 1988. The two leading providers of

Table 12.1 Referral guidelines to chiropractors.

Appropriate conditions for referrals	Inappropriate conditions for referrals
Mechanical low back pain	Cauda equina syndrome
Mild-moderate disc lesion	Organic referred back pain
Poor posture	Connective tissue disorders
Deconditioned spines	Inflammatory arthritis
Acute cervical torticollis	Advanced osteoporosis
Post-traumatic soft tissue injuries	Spinal tumours
Back pain in pregnancy	Spinal metastases
Post-natal back pain	Suspected infection
Cervicogenic headaches	Cervical spine instability
Back strains/sprains from sports injury	Evidence of spinal cord injury

ABC of Spinal Disorders. Edited by Andrew Clarke, Alwyn Jones, Michael O'Malley and Robert McLaren.
© 2010 by Blackwell Publishing, ISBN: 978-1-4051-7069-7.

mainstream chiropractic education in the United Kingdom are the Anglo-European College of Chiropractic (Bournemouth University) and the Welsh Institute of Chiropractic (University of Glamorgan). Both provide a minimum 4-year undergraduate programme leading to a BSc (Hons) or Masters award in Chiropractic but are also involved in postgraduate Masters and PhD programmes.

The course content is similar in many respects to conventional medical training, with anatomy, physiology and biochemistry forming the core of the undergraduate curriculum in the early years. Emphasis is placed on neurology, neuroanatomy, biomechanics and general medical diagnosis as the course progresses and, as one might expect, manual skills are taught from the outset. Chiropractors also undergo training in radiology and radiography, and are thus qualified to both take and read X-rays upon graduation.

To qualify for membership of the British Chiropractic Association, new graduate chiropractors must undertake a pre-registration training programme during their first postgraduate year where they are under the supervision of an approved clinical trainer. All chiropractors in the United Kingdom are required to undertake continuing professional development (CPD) and submit an annual return to the GCC demonstrating evidence of postgraduate studies and learning cycles.

The College of Chiropractors is an apolitical organization that provides postgraduate training to chiropractors and complements the roles of the professional organizations. It has more than 1500 members in the United Kingdom and produces the journal *Clinical Chiropractic*.

Chiropractors qualified overseas must take and successfully pass a GCC Test of Competence before being eligible to practice as a chiropractor in the United Kingdom. This test examines proficiency and competence in a range of assessment, clinical and diagnostic areas of practice.

Chiropractic assessment

Chiropractors are primary health-care practitioners and therefore have a duty to undertake a full medical history when assessing patients. In addition to obtaining details on the chief complaint, chiropractors will also obtain detailed medical information to determine the health status of the patient; this will include details on current and previous medical conditions, medication, occupational and lifestyle factors and previous medical history. During this process, chiropractors will often identify other medical issues, which may be impacting upon or causing spinal pain, enabling prompt and appropriate onward referral to be made.

Chiropractors undertake a careful postural inspection and perform standard orthopaedic and neurological examinations of the spine. Their extensive training in manual palpation skills means that they are able to detect often subtle areas of mechanical restriction in the spinal joints and related structures; some chiropractors refer to these areas of restriction as fixations or subluxations.

As chiropractic treatment often involves the use of manual therapy techniques, it is important that chiropractors ensure that treatment can be safely undertaken. For this reason, chiropractors may utilize further investigations, which may include diagnostic imaging in the form of X-ray or magnetic resonance imaging (MRI).

Many UK chiropractors are qualified to both take and read plain X-rays.

Chiropractic diagnosis of spinal disorders utilizes a conventional triage of mechanical spinal pain, nerve root pain or serious spinal pathology, with sub-classifications for each group. Typically mechanical back pain will arise from disorders of the facet joints, sacroiliac joints or spinal soft tissues; nerve root pain from disc lesions or from lateral or central stenosis; and serious pathology from tumours, infections or fractures. In addition to this, chiropractors will also consider biopsychosocial factors that may impact on a patient's likely response to pain and disability.

Chiropractors use terminology common to other health professionals specializing in spinal disorders, but like all medical specialities, some words, phrases and notations are peculiar to chiropractic – manipulation is often referred to as spinal **adjustment**, lesions are known as **subluxations** or **fixations**, and misalignments in the spine may be recorded to as **listings**.

Chiropractors are encouraged to communicate their findings to the patient's GP and other members of the clinical team. Such an approach enables them to participate fully in clinical decision-making and places patients at the heart of the treatment process. Increasingly, through adopting this integrated approach to care, chiropractors are fast-becoming part of the mainstream musculoskeletal team.

Treatment techniques

Contrary to the popular belief that chiropractic treatment consists solely of spinal manipulation, it is important to understand that chiropractic is a package of care, which involves providing advice, reassurance, exercise and rehabilitation as well as manual therapies (spinal manipulation, stretching techniques and soft tissue mobilization). As primary healthcare providers, chiropractors are well qualified to determine which treatment is likely to provide most benefit under the circumstances of the case.

Chiropractors are among the most highly trained in spinal manipulation, which is taught intensively throughout the 4-year undergraduate programme. Spinal manipulation is not new – there is evidence of it having been used for thousands of years – but modern chiropractic techniques are safe, effective and specific. It is also evidence-based and has been included in treatment guidelines, particularly for the management of low back pain.

While there are a number of spinal manipulative techniques available, which may use manual skills or the application of force using an instrument, common to all is the objective of mobilizing specific areas of vertebral or pelvic joint restriction. Technique selection depends on the physical characteristics of the patient, the diagnosis and practitioner preference.

Subscribing to the evidence supporting an active care approach to spinal disorders, many chiropractors advocate spinal rehabilitation programmes. Often using facilities within their clinics, chiropractors offer supervised programmes of exercise to develop strength, stamina, endurance and balance. Particularly effective for chronic low back pain and whiplash associated disorders, supervised strengthening and rehabilitation programmes are consistent with an evidenced approach to the management of spinal disorders and is an important component of the overall care package.

Safety

Chiropractic treatment is safe in the hands of registered practitioners and reports of serious adverse events are rare. Mild side effects from certain types of treatment are, however, quite common and short-term muscle stiffness and post-manipulative soreness can be expected, although these tend to disappear within 48 hours. Before treatment, patients are informed of the known risks and benefits of care and it is ensured that full informed consent is obtained.

Spinal manipulation is not suitable for all and chiropractors should be sure that tissues can withstand manipulation before it is performed. Contraindications to spinal manipulation include cauda equina syndrome, advanced osteoporosis, malignant disease, conditions which involve vascular fragility, possible fracture sites and rare connective tissue disorders.

Chiropractic spinal manipulation has in the past been associated with stroke and artery dissection and this has fuelled speculation that manipulation of the neck should not be performed. However, independent research published in 2008 by the Task Force on Neck Pain and its Associated Disorders indicated that the risk of stroke after visiting a chiropractor was no higher than that after visiting a GP. This compelling study supports the view that chiropractic manipulation of the neck is not only safe, but may be the treatment of choice for mechanical neck pain.

In the area of the lower back, complications of spinal manipulation are very rare. Reviews have demonstrated that the risk of cauda equina syndrome being caused by spinal manipulation is extremely low, even in the presence of a prolapsed intervertebral disc. As with the cervical spine, manipulation of the lower back may cause temporary mild effects of stiffness and aching, although these generally subside within 48 hours.

Referring to a chiropractor

The GMC's *Good Medical Practice* (*2006*) document deals with referral and delegation. Because regulated health professionals are accountable to a statutory regulatory body (the GCC), chiropractors may receive referrals from their medical colleagues. GPs are therefore able to employ, contract the services of, or make referrals to chiropractors with full confidence that their patients are protected by statutory health-care regulation.

Useful addresses

British Chiropractic Association, 59 Castle Street, Reading RG1 7SN
Tel. 0118 950 5950 www.chiropractic-uk.co.uk
College of Chiropractors, Chiltern Chambers, 37 St Peters Avenue, Reading RG4 7DH Tel. 0118 946 9730 www.colchiro.org.uk
General Chiropractic Council, 44 Wicklow Street, London WC1X 9HL
Tel. 0207 713 5155 www.gcc-uk.org

Further reading

Cassidy JD, Boyle E, Cote P, He Y, Hogg-Johnson S, Silver FL, Bondy SJ *et al*. Risk of vertebrobasilar stroke and chiropractic care: results of a population-based case-control and case-crossover study. *Spine* 2008 Feb 15; **33**(4 Suppl): S176–S183.

Department of Health. *The Musculoskeletal Services Framework. A Joint Responsibility: Doing It Differently*. Department of Health, 2006.

General Chiropractic Council. *Code of Practice and Standard of Proficiency* 4th edition. General Chiropractic Council, 2010 (Effective from 30 June 2010).

General Medical Council (2006). *Good Medical Practice*. General Medical Council, 2006.

National Institute for Health and Clinical Excellence. *Low Back Pain: Early Management of Persistent Non-specific Low Back Pain*. National Institute for Health and Clinical Excellence, 2009.

UK BEAM Trial Team. The UK Back Pain Exercise and Manipulation (BEAM) randomised trial: cost effectiveness of physical treatments for back pain in primary care. *British Medical Journal* 2004; **329**(7479): 1377.

CHAPTER 13

Pain Management

Darryl Johnston

Royal Devon and Exeter Hospital, Devon, UK

OVERVIEW

- Pain management is a multimodal discipline that includes self-help
- Evaluation and education are fundamentals to good pain management
- In severe pain, a stepwise approach to analgesia is advocated
- Total resolution of pain may not be possible without any intervention
- Avoidance of chronicity and dependence is a key aim of treatment

---

Back pain is very common in the developed world affecting approximately 70% of the population at some point in their life, only 1 to 2% will have a serious spinal pathology. Generally, the condition is self-limiting, but may reoccur in as many as 50%. The disability that develops as a consequence of back pain is well documented and the cost to society is ever increasing. In 1998, the direct cost of health care was estimated at £1632 million and accounts for 4% of GP consultations. Almost all acute back pain is managed in primary care.

Assessment

Serious pathology must first be excluded (red flags). The remaining patients can be reassured. Patients can be assessed for psychosocial risk factors (yellow flags) that make them more likely to go on to develop chronic pain (pain lasting longer than 3 months). The degree of distress and disability that is caused by back pain should also be noted. There is no relationship between the severity of pain and the disability it causes. The patient must be individually treated in an attempt to reduce disability. Finally it should be noted whether nerve root pain is present.

Management

A management plan should be set up between the doctor and patient. The patient can be given educational advice as to what to

---

ABC of Spinal Disorders. Edited by Andrew Clarke, Alwyn Jones, Michael O'Malley and Robert McLaren.
© 2010 by Blackwell Publishing, ISBN: 978-1-4051-7069-7.

---

expect over the next few weeks and what they can do to improve their symptoms.

Unreasonable expectations must be ruled out and inappropriate fears and beliefs dismissed. Information leaflets are an ideal way of passing on this information whilst reinforcing the message from the doctor.

A review date can be made when the patient and doctor can discuss the progress made and allow for change of the management according to results. It must be made clear that if their symptoms change or significantly worsen they must come for review earlier.

Daily activities must be continued as much as possible and patients should be encouraged to return to work. Randomized control trials have now shown that continuing daily activity at best will speed up recovery from symptoms and at worst will have no effect on recovery time. It will also help prevent the progression to chronic disability.

Self-help should be encouraged at every opportunity. There are a myriad of techniques and programmes advocated by health-care providers and patients themselves. Commonly used ones include McKenzie Technique, Pilates Method and the Alexander Technique.

A New Zealand physiotherapist, Robin McKenzie, published a book entitled 'Treat Your Own Back' in 1980. On page 1 he pointed out that you, as the back pain sufferer, are responsible for the management of your back. He felt that self-help is more effective in the long-term treatment of back pain. The book provides education about the nature of the problem and a series of exercises to improve it.

Pilates Method was introduced during the First World War by Joseph Pilates, as a rehabilitation programme for the servicemen. He called his technique **Contrology**, believing very fervently in the intimate relationship between physical and mental health. The key principles of Pilates are harmony between the mind and body by breathing, centreing, concentration, control, precision and flow of movement.

The Alexander technique was developed by Frederick Alexander. He was an actor, who kept losing his voice. The medical profession was unable to find an obvious reason therefore, he took it upon himself to seek one. Alexander, with the use of mirrors, found that he stiffened his body. His studies led to developing a technique to improve posture and movement. It is a technique that is taught by a coach, but then undertaken by patients themselves. There are conflicting reports as to its efficacy.

Finally, encouraging physical exercise to improve general fitness should be explored. In 2005, Hurwitz et al., found that general programmes were linked to improvements but specific back exercises were not. The benefits of exercise are both physical and psychological to the participant. However, it can be difficult to persuade patients to undertake exercise, because of their fears of pain exacerbation. In 1999, Keen et al., reported that the perception of pain returning and avoidance behaviour were the main reasons influencing physical exercise in patients with low back pain.

Bed rest has been shown to have a poor effect on recovery and in trials it has been shown to decrease recovery rate and increase time to resuming normal daily activities. In addition, bed rest leads to joint stiffness, muscle wasting, loss of bone mineral density and increases the incidence of venous thromboembolism.

Cold packs or low-level heat wraps have also been shown to provide symptomatic relief but only in the short term.

Transcutaneous electrical nerve stimulation (TENS) machines and spinal manipulation have not been shown to have any effect on acute back pain.

Pharmacological interventions

These are given to relieve the symptoms of pain.

Simple back pain

Paracetamol is the first-line simple analgesic used for mild to moderate pain and should be used regularly together with a non-steroidal anti-inflammatory drug (NSAID) such as voltarol or ibuprofen provided there are no contraindications. For more severe musculoskeletal pain codeine or tramadol can be added; if used regularly a laxative may also be needed.

Nerve root pain (leg pain and buttock pain)

Paracetamol is again the first-line analgesic. NSAIDs are then the second-line analgesics but have been shown not to be very effective in relieving radicular pain in some studies. Stronger opioids have also been shown not to be as effective on radicular pain and they should only be considered when all other measures fail.

Review

Traditionally, patients are reviewed after 4 to 6 weeks.

Patients showing signs of improvement can be given further advice and reassurance, but those patients showing no signs of improvement or deterioration need to have every aspect of their management reassessed. Red flags need to be again excluded and the presence of nerve root pain assessed. If there is no improvement to nerve root pain then a referral to a specialist should be made. An adjustment of their medication can also be made to control their symptoms, either increasing their analgesia, or adding an adjunct such as an antidepressant or anticonvulsant.

Amitryptylline is a commonly used antidepressant, which is an effective analgesic and sedative and for that reason is given at night in small doses. It can take 2 to 3 days to be fully effective; therefore, it is started early in pain management.

There is conflicting evidence in regards to the use of muscle relaxants (e.g. Diazepam). If there are symptoms of muscle spasm the relaxants can be used, but only a short course is recommended as they can lead to dependence. Side effects are also common such as drowsiness and dizziness and patients must be warned not to drive for the next 24 hours after stopping these drugs.

Adjuncts such as anticonvulsants and antidepressants can be very effective in the treatment of radicular pain but do not work immediately. A first-line treatment would be to add either an antidepressant or an anticonvulsant. Amitryptylline is the antidepressant of choice. Gabapentin and/or pregabalin are anticonvulsants and are also very effective in treating neuropathic pain and have the additional advantages of enhancing mood and improving sleep patterns. Their main disadvantages are that they do not work immediately. Pregabalin is newer and faster acting. If the patient fails to respond to one adjunct, the next line of treatment would be to use both an antidepressant and an anticonvulsant. The final step in the ladder would be to add in a strong opioid, but nerve root pain only partially responds to stronger opioids.

The impact that back pain is having on daily activities must also be assessed. The patient can be formally assessed for risk factors in chronic pain, that is, the presence of Yellow flags. 'Yellow flags' include various psychological and social factors that lead to a negative perception of what they are going through. A specialist centre can assess these patients suitability for cognitive behavioural therapy and biopsychosocial assessment. This will often involve assessment by a physiotherapist and a clinical psychologist who can then decide if the patient would respond better to a more structured programme such as 'back school', where exercise routines and coping strategies are reinforced, or whether they require a more individual approach.

Cognitive behavioural therapy, supervised exercise therapy, educational interventions and multidisciplinary (biopsychosocial) treatment have a role in the treatment of back pain, both in those in whom the prognostic markers (yellow flags) indicate are at risk from developing long-term disability and also in those who do not respond to more conventional therapy.

Further reading

Bigos S, Bowyer O, Braen G et al. Acute Low Back Pain in Adults. Clinical practice guidelines no. 14. AHCPR publication no. 95-0642. Agency for health care policy and research, Public health Service, US department of health and Human Services, Rockville, MD, 1994.

Hurwitz EL, Morgenstern H, Chiao C. Effects of recreational physical activity and back exercises on low back pain and psychological distress: findings from the UCLA low back pain study. American Journal of Public Health 2005; 95(10): 1817–1822.

Keen S et al. Individuals with low back pain: how do they view physical activity? Family Practice 1999; 16(1): 39–45.

Maurits VT, Annette B, Trudy B et al. on behalf of the COST B13 Working Group on Guidelines for the Management of Acute Low Back Pain in Primary Care. European Guidelines for the Management of Acute Nonspecific Low Back pain in Primary Care.

McKenzie R. Treat Your Own Back. Spinal Publications, New Zealand, 1980.

Nadler SF, Steiner DJ, Erasala GN et al. Continuous low level heat wrap therapy provides more efficacy than ibuprofen and acetaminophen for acute low back pain. Spine 2002; 27: 1012–1017.

Royal College of General Practitioners. *Clinical Guidelines for the Management of Acute Low Back Pain*. London, UK, 1996 and 1999.

Van Tulder MW, Esmail R, Bombardier C *et al.* NSAIDS for non-specific low back pain (Cochrane review). In: *The Cochrane Library*, Issue 4. Update software, Oxford, 2000.

Waddell G. *The Back Pain Revolution*. 2nd edn. Churchill Livingstone, Edinburgh, 2004.

Waddell G, Feder G, Lewis M. Systematic reviews of bed rest and advice to stay active for acute low back pain. *British Journal of General Practice* 1997; **47**: 647–652.

CHAPTER 14

Psychological Approaches to Managing Chronic Back Pain

Elenor McLaren[1] and Robert McLaren[2]

[1]Clinical Psychologist, Charing Cross Hospital, London, UK
[2]General Practitioner, London, UK

OVERVIEW

- Encourage a 'self-management' approach rather than cure seeking

- Educate about 'pacing' activities

- 'Goal setting' – short and long term – towards valued areas

- Highlight thinking traps and teach patients to question thoughts

- 'Mindfulness' and changing the focus of attention can aid pain management

---

Introduction

The experience of chronic pain is more than a sensory experience – it affects many areas of life including social, occupational and emotional functioning. Psychological approaches to managing chronic pain consider these areas.

Patients have frequently tried a range of medical approaches with limited long-term gains and can become trapped in a cycle of cure-seeking behaviour. This chapter briefly discusses techniques that can help patients discover this and enable them to make the paradigm shift from cure seeking to self-management. While it is unrealistic for clinicians to use all of these techniques in a primary care setting, being aware of them will enable the clinicians to promote and reinforce the self-management message.

The techniques help people appreciate that pain is an emotional as well as a sensory experience. It is useful first to explore with individuals the impact pain has had on their lives. Two exercises may help: 'The Rolling Snow Ball Exercise' and 'The Struggle with Pain Exercise' (McCracken, 2005) (Figures 14.1 and 14.2).

These exercises can help patients realize that the struggle to try to cure pain can add to their suffering more than it lessens it and actually moves them away from the things they value in life. Difficulties with this paradigm shift tend to be the largest obstacle to self-management. Once the shift is made, many experience improvements in their quality of life.

ABC of Spinal Disorders. Edited by Andrew Clarke, Alwyn Jones, Michael O'Malley and Robert McLaren.
© 2010 by Blackwell Publishing, ISBN: 978-1-4051-7069-7.

Activity pacing and goal setting
Pacing

- Chronic pain (and fatigue) patients can become caught in a trap of **activity cycling**: doing a lot on 'good days' when the pain is less and then doing little on 'bad days' (which inevitably follow good days because too much has been done). Over time activity cycling tends to lead to people doing less and less. It becomes more difficult for patients to plan because they don't know how they will be; they worry about letting others down and others may eventually expect less of them and may take things over for them . . .

- Activity cycling can be overcome through learning PACING (Table 14.1) – being able to do some activities daily without making the pain worse. It involves establishing a regular manageable amount of activity based on a plan and **not** how the person feels that day. The plan should be aimed at what can be expected with a tolerable amount of pain rather than when pain-free or in agony. Often it takes some trial and error to get the optimal starting amount.

Short-term goal setting

- Goal setting enables people to take back some control over their activities and pain.

- Completed goals promote a sense of purpose and achievement by signposting progression in physical and mental activity.

- Short-term goals should be SMART (Table 14.2).

Long-term goal setting based on 'valued directions'

- It is helpful to get people to think about the valued directions in their life that are important to them (e.g. being a loving

Table 14.1 A way to plan regular manageable activities for patients with chronic pain.

PACING: Activities need to be:
Broken down into smaller tasks and *priorities established*
Done using a *'little and often'* approach, allowing a *regular change in position*
Based on a *baseline time* that is manageable even when in pain (e.g. walking for 10 minutes)
Increased gradually by planning a realistic build-up rate
Time-limited: people need to be encouraged to stick to what they had planned and *avoid the '5 minutes more syndrome'* even if they feel good

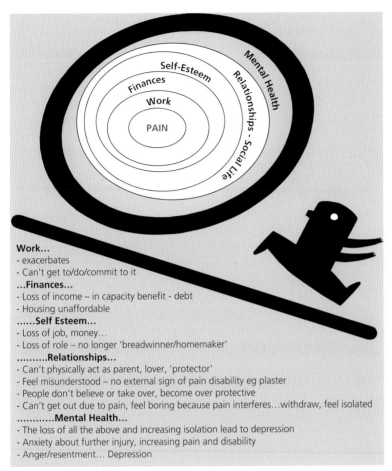

Work...
- exacerbates
- Can't get to/do/commit to it
...Finances...
- Loss of income – in capacity benefit - debt
- Housing unaffordable
......Self Esteem...
- Loss of job, money...
- Loss of role – no longer 'breadwinner/homemaker'
..........Relationships...
- Can't physically act as parent, lover, 'protector'
- Feel misunderstood – no external sign of pain disability eg plaster
- People don't believe or take over, become over protective
- Can't get out due to pain, feel boring because pain interferes...withdraw, feel isolated
............Mental Health...
- The loss of all the above and increasing isolation lead to depression
- Anxiety about further injury, increasing pain and disability
- Anger/resentment... Depression

Figure 14.1 The Rolling Snowball Exercise – with the patient construct a snow ball where you put the pain in the middle and add concentric circles pertaining to effects pain has had on their lives. Pictorially then the pain experience becomes much bigger than just the medical aspect. It helps patients to see the effect of pain is multifactorial and therefore they need to take a multifactorial approach to managing it.

What have you tried	Short-term results	Long-term results	What does your experience tell you?
To reduce or control your pain and other symptoms?	Were the symptoms reduced?	Did you move closer to the way you want to live your life?	

Figure 14.2 The 'Struggle with Pain Exercise' (McCracken, 2005) – helps patients to discover that while medical interventions sometimes help in the short term, they often do not cure the pain long term and that constantly seeking medical cures can impede them from getting on with their lives and managing their chronic pain optimally.

Table 14.2 A way to set appropriate goals with people with chronic pain.

SMART goal setting

Specific:	What exactly does the person want to do?
Measurable:	How far? How long? How often?
Achievable:	Realistic?
Relevant:	Setting their own goals – not those others want them to do
Time-limited:	When by? Need to set a realistic time scale

partner/parent, being successful at their job . . .). What would they like written on their epitaph? Few wish for 'he/she spent much of his/her life fighting chronic pain'! (McCracken, 2005)

- Get people to set long-term goals around their valued directions. Encourage people to engage with such long-term goals, and help them to identify areas of personal growth and the activities that are important to them with family, friends and work. They will need to balance these against the degree of pain, aversive emotions and/or discouraging thoughts they are prepared to tolerate.
- Focusing on pursuing valued directions gives people rationale/motivation to learn to self-manage chronic pain. When people get trapped in the struggle to cure their pain, they can often lose sight of the things that matter to them.

Table 14.3 A method for those with chronic pain to evaluate and challenge upsetting (and often unhelpful) thoughts.

Systemic method for evaluation upsetting thoughts
• Do they help me?
• Do I have any evidence to support these thoughts?
• What would a friend say in this situation?
• How would I have viewed this situation before I had a pain problem?
• What can I do to change my situation?
It can be helpful for people to write down their thoughts and consider more alternative helpful ways of looking at their situation: Barrier thought *vs.* Alternatives that promote my goal

Managing thoughts and behaviour
The impacts of thoughts

- It is helpful to educate people about the cognitive behavioural model where thoughts and behaviours impact how you feel physically and emotionally. This can be illustrated using their own examples.
- It can be fruitful to introduce people to common 'thinking traps', which include catastrophizing, all or no thinking, disqualifying the positive, jumping to conclusions, emotional reasoning and personalization using their examples (Beck, 1979).
- Teach them a systematic method for evaluating upsetting thoughts (Table 14.3).

Habits and pain behaviours – The impact of chronic pain on relationships

- Chronic pain often has a negative impact on people's relationships particularly where unwelcome role change/loss has occurred.
- Communication and anger management skills can help with this. Getting people to express their needs assertively rather than aggressively/passively often involves a change in the choice of language, timing and body language – all of which can be learnt.
- It is important for people to accept that they will have more success with working on changing themselves than trying to change others.

Working with obstacles: a problem solving technique

The technique is simple and effective – easily dismissed as too simple. Most people use parts of it without being aware of it (Figure 14.3).

Techniques to manage pain, stress and discomfort
Attentional focus and mindfulness

- Various exercises can be useful in illustrating to the patients the power of attention in the pain experience and how people can have more control over where and how they focus their attention than they think.

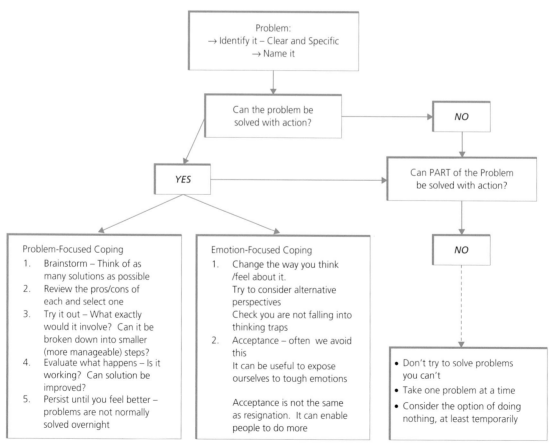

Figure 14.3 Problem solving – using problem- and emotion-focused techniques. These concepts are from Lazarus and Folkman, 2005.

- Kabat-Zinn's (1990) definition of mindfulness – 'paying attention in a particular way: on purpose, in the present moment, and non-judgementally' provides a different way of experiencing everyday activities such as eating, driving and so on. It demonstrates to people how much of their time is spent in 'automatic pilot' which can consist of (without people realizing) self-defeating patterns of behaviour and thinking.

Progressive muscular relaxation

- Muscle tension and anxiety/stress can increase a person's experience of pain. Having chronic pain can make dealing with life stresses harder; therefore, having several ways of coping with stress is important.
- Progressive muscular relaxation (PMR) can help people cope with pain by reducing muscle tension and anxiety/stress. It can also give people space to notice thoughts, feelings and reactions which may be increasing their suffering.
- PMR involves tensing and then relaxing muscle groups in a systematic manner noting the different associated sensations whilst focusing on abdominal breathing.

The body scan

- An exercise in formal mindfulness that takes approximately 45 minutes and becomes more useful the more it is practised. (Kabat-Zinn, 1990)
- Lie down on your back in a comfortable/warm place. Close your eyes gently, feel the rising and falling of your belly with each breath, take a few moments to feel your body as a whole, the places where you are in contact with the floor/bed, then bring attention to toes of left foot and see if you can direct or channel your breathing into them as if you are breathing 'in to and **from**' your toes. Focus on the sensations you feel or do not feel in that area . . . then progress on up the foot . . . ankle . . . leg etc.

Table 14.4 Planning for pain flare-ups in advance enables patients to retain a sense of control.

Plan for tackling flare-ups	
Pain relief:	How much and when? When to visit a GP/chemist etc?
Activity pacing:	Cut activities by half and return to them in 1 week
Relaxation:	How and when?
Communication:	What and how will you tell other people during a flare-up? What do you need them to do?
Thinking:	During a flare-up I will remind myself that I have had this problem before and I coped with it then and I can cope with it now

GP, general practitioner.

- Attention will wander; just focus on getting it back to breathing 'into' parts of the body.
- Tapes are available to help with this type of exercise.
- Can be done with eyes open if subject keeps falling asleep.
- Can be useful where pain prevents PMR.

Working with flare-ups

- Flare-ups when the pain increases for 2 days or more. It is helpful to plan in advance how to deal with these – Table 14.4.

Further reading

Beck AT, Rush AJ, Shaw BF & Emery G. *Cognitive Therapy of Depression.* Guildford, New York, 1979.

Kabat-Zinn J. *Full Catastrophe Living; The Programme of the Stress Reduction Clinic at the University of Massachusetts Medical Centre.* Dell, New York, USA, 1990.

Lazarus RS, Folkman S. *Stress, Appraisal and Coping.* Springer, New York, 1984.

McCracken LM. *Contextual Cognitive Behavioural Therapy for Chronic Pain.* ISAP Press, Seattle, WA, 2005.

Index

Note: page numbers in *italics* refer to figures, those in **bold** refer to tables and boxes

ABC of Skin Cancer

Edited by Sajjad Rajpar & Jerry Marsden
Sandwell & West Birmingham NHS Trust; Selly Oak Hospital, Birmingham

- A new, highly illustrated, concise, factual, and practical overview of skin cancers and pre-cancerous lesions
- Focuses on diagnosis, differential diagnosis, common pitfalls, and outlines best practice management in primary care
- In line with the latest NICE guidelines in the UK, places the emphasis on the pivotal role that GPs play in the screening, diagnosis and referral of skin cancers and pre-cancerous lesions
- Also includes chapters on non-surgical treatment and prevention

April 2008 | 9781405162197 | 80 pages | £19.99/$39.95/€24.90

ABC of Clinical Electrocardiography
SECOND EDITION

Edited by Francis Morris, William Brady & John Camm
Northern General Hospital, Sheffield; University of Virginia Health Sciences Centre, Charlottesville; St. George's University of London

- A new edition of this practical guide to the interpretation of ECGs for the non-specialist
- The ABC format lends itself to clearly illustrate full 12-lead ECGs
- Sets out the main patterns seen in cardiac disorders in clinical practice, covering the fundamentals of interpretation and analysis
- Covers exercise tolerance testing and provides clear anatomical illustrations to explain key points

May 2008 | 9781405170642 | 112 pages | £26.99/$49.95/€34.90

ABC of Complementary Medicine
SECOND EDITION

Edited by Catherine Zollman, Andrew J. Vickers & Janet Richardson
General Practitioner, Bristol; Memorial Sloan-Kettering Cancer Center, New York; University of Plymouth

- This thoroughly revised and updated second edition offers an authoritative introduction to complementary therapies
- Includes the latest information on efficacy of treatments
- Places a new emphasis in patient management
- Ideal guide for primary care practitioners

June 2008 | 9781405136570 | 64 pages | £21.99/$40.95/€27.90

ABC of Eating Disorders

Edited by Jane Morris
Royal Edinburgh Hospital

- Charts the diagnosis of different eating disorders and their management and treatment by GPs, dieticians and psychiatrists
- Examines diagnosis, management and treatment by health professionals and through self-help
- Helps primary care practitioners recognise eating disorders in young people presenting with other problems
- Supports the work of general psychiatrists and physicians, community health teams and teaching staff
- Includes medico-legal aspects of treating eating disorders and specialist referral

August 2008 | 9780727918437 | 80 pages | £19.99/$35.95/€24.90

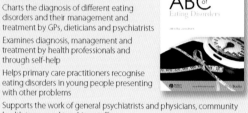

ABC of Tubes, Drains, Lines and Frames

Edited by Adam Brooks, Peter F. Mahoney & Brian Rowlands
Queen's Medical Centre, University of Nottingham; The Royal Centre for Defence Medicine; The Royal Centre for Defence Medicine

- A brand new title in the *ABC* series
- A full-colour, practical guide to the key issues involved in the assessment and management of surgical adjuncts
- Covers the care of post-operative patients in primary care
- Highlights common pitfalls and includes "trouble shooting" sections

October 2008 | 9781405160148 | 88 pages | £19.99/$35.95/€24.90

ABC of Headache

Edited by Anne MacGregor & Alison Frith
Both The City of London Migraine Clinic

- Uses real case histories to guide the reader through symptoms to diagnosis and management or, where relevant, to specialist referral
- A highly illustrated, informative and practical source of knowledge and offers links to further information and resources
- An essential guide for healthcare professionals, at all levels of training, looking for possible causes of presenting symptoms of headache

October 2008 | 9781405170666 | 88 pages | £19.99/$35.95/€24.90

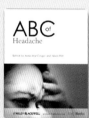